HAPPY *healthy* THYROID

The Essential Steps
to Healing Naturally

by Andrea Beaman, HHC, AADP

HAPPY, HEALTHY, THYROID

Cover design Julie Mueller
jam graphics & design, llc

WHAT PEOPLE ARE SAYING

Finally, we have a voice in the crowd that speaks loud and clear and most importantly truthful about our health. With her matter of fact common sense, based on experience, she guides the way to better health.

I am 64 years young and was diagnosed with hypothyroidism at 18. For years I was on synthroid and at 50 I said no more. For the last decade I had been experimenting with herbs, acupuncture, diet and exercise, naturopathic systems and so forth to find the answers to feeling good and live a vibrant life.

Andrea started with one thing that struck me dumbfounded... chew your food, take time. Sounds simple enough. Wait until your practice it.
I realized I was an unconscious eater...just going through the motions and never being aware, always multitasking or being social while eating and never just being with my food. This alone was worth taking the class as it has helped this emotional eater put on the breaks and begin to eat consciously. I feel a relationship between my food and my body. This was the beginning of wellness for me.

Be prepared Andrea is going to shake up your world. So much information and wisdom, fresh new ideas, science that works, and life skills that create change. I feel better everyday due to Andrea's teaching. A positive solution to living a life well lived. Thank you, Andrea. — *Deborah Kelly*

My doctor wanted to put me on medication immediately and I decided to wait and see if it could heal itself with Andrea's recommendations and her Nourishing Thyroid program. I loved the way she helped me, the way she teaches and the recommendations she gave us really worked out for me. My last blood test was great, my TSH levels not only where normal, they were better than ever, as the number was increasing the past few years, and this time is perfect! I am so happy with the course and I will try to keep doing all the things I have learned. Within only 4 months I got my TSH levels perfect, without any medication, only following Andrea's suggestions, increasing my resting time, meditating, having good quality foods, introducing seaweeds to my diet, and finding out my truth. I encourage anyone to do the course, it helped my health and in my case not only this, it also inspired me! Thanks Andrea. — *Laura Llacuna*

The content Andrea provided was very helpful. I eat most of her recipes, and keep in mind her suggestions. She has encouraged me to stay strong, not get caught up in what others say and doctors tell me. I was able to heal my thyroid without radiation or any medication. — *Sharon Siodmak*

Andrea's in-depth knowledge of thyroid disease and oriental diagnosis when way beyond anything I was taught and learned prior to her class in a meaningful, natural, and sustainable way. Andrea's knowledge has been really so helpful, and I have picked up some of the missing information pieces that I needed for my health. Andrea suggested some bone broth. Well, I did not realize how impactful that would become. A simple thing like chicken broth with chicken and veggies made me feel more balanced than ever and not crave sugar in any form. I eat chicken and veggies all the time, but the broth was the real key. Who would have thought! WOW, major, major accomplishment. I feel blessed to have found and met her. Thank you Andrea!!! You are like a rare pearl! — *Joan Ungerleider*

Andrea's enthusiasm and positive attitude is very motivational. The new information I learned was valuable and Andrea's presentations helped to clarify information I was conflicted about and reinforced my commitment to eat healthy, whole foods. One of the most helpful things I learned about was nightshade vegetables and their effect on the thyroid. — *Anne Parrish*

The biggest lesson I learned was you are in control if you listen to what your body is telling you. If you crave meat eat it (I was a vegetarian for a while) and if you crave vegetables eat them. You know your body better than anyone - including your doctor. I thought I was eating healthy but it turns out the foods I was eating were not good for my thyroid. I was one of those who had a green shake with fruit, raw kale, coconut water and spinach every morning and was running 2-3 miles 5-6 times a week. It turns out that is not what my body needs. I can't wait to take my learning one step further. — *Cindy Sullivan*

Andrea's Nourishing Thyroid Health Class was exactly what I needed to move forward with the healing of my thyroid. She started out with the small, yet big things to be aware of everyday to make a big difference in our free radical consumption and digestion health. Who would have thought that many of us have forgotten to chew, smell, and taste our food? She teaches us to honor and create a spiritual connection with our hurried lives and promote change.

I have learned so much about my thyroid, things I wish I knew a decade ago. I am in gratitude for the recipes, action guides. Thank you for the promotion of awareness toward our big beautiful world of local plants and animals that provide us with our nutrition. I feel healthier overall, more energy, more awareness of what my body reacts to, and the ability to love myself when I need a restorative time rather than a place of action. I make time to breath deeply in this time and oxygenate my physical body and cleanse my spiritual one.

Andrea has opened my world to embrace my autoimmune disease and live a better quality of life, knowing how to feed, love and heal it. It is very refreshing to see the new content added to our tool boxes as Andrea continues her education and understanding of the world around her. She truly is the example of the ever-evolving educator combining all her knowledge to promote health to the world and herself. Just watch a video of her smiling face as it is clear she loves her life and calling, a wonderful mentor to the world of healing. Thank you Andrea — *Brenda Young*

When I was diagnosed with thyroid and diabetes I researched everything and re-tooled my kitchen accordingly. But, in all of these years, I never knew the whole story on grains. I first read about proper grain preparation in Andrea's cookbook, but then the first module expanded on that information. I also never realized the benefits of bone broth. Not only is it good for the thyroid but is also beneficial for my blood sugars as well. And I love that I no longer have waste from my poultry and meat dishes. I keep everything in plastic zip locks in the freezer so it is ready when I have time to make more. It's so convenient to pull out a serving of broth when I'm in a hurry or just not hungry for a full meal. The bonus module with pharmacist Karyn Bender was fantastic. I've been taking a very low dose of Levothyroxine for 9 months and just now started to develop fatigue around mid afternoon. I thought it might be iron deficient related but not sure. I would drink some bone broth and would feel better. Then I learned that Levothyroxine can affect iron absorption even from a multi-vitamin. Since I took both the med early in the morning and the vitamin an hour later with breakfast I changed to taking the vitamin at dinner time. Mid afternoon fatigue is gone! — *Tina Rengel*

There is so much conflicting and confusing advice out there and Andrea simplified it and made it really easy to understand. Andrea's personable manner really motivated me to change my diet. I added seaweed to my diet. I would have never thought to do that. – *Sadiyya Patel*

To hear what other folks are saying go to
AndreaBeaman.com/Thyroid

ACKNOWLEDGMENTS

From my mother's battle with breast cancer to my own thyroid disease, each illness that has come into my life has proved to be a blessing. These medical conditions have taught me new aspects about healing the body from an alternative point of view. Every day, I give thanks to my beautiful thyroid gland for helping me discover new and more healthful ways to exist in the world. The greatest thing I've discovered is that the thyroid is my emotional and spiritual connection to voicing my truth in a healthful way. This book is the expression of that voice. Thyroid disease has become my personal catalyst to discovering my life's work: teaching and sharing knowledge, and for that I am forever grateful.

I wouldn't be able to share knowledge in an effective way if it weren't for the people closest to me who free up my time and energy, so I can continue creating great content to share with the world. It's hard work running a business, and it simply cannot be done well without an *exceptional* team to take care of the details. Amanda Manganaro and Erica Swammy are that core team for me. Thank you ladies for all of your hard work and dedication. I appreciate your work every day—even on the days we are not working!

Writing a book is like having a baby. The idea for the book is planted in the mind, it is then nourished and developed for a period of time, and when ready, it is brought out into the world for everyone else to see. Ahhhhh yes, such a beautiful little book baby! I couldn't have birthed this book without the support and expertise of Paula Jacobson and Sheilah Kaufman. Their tag-team editing skills kept the content flowing and growing beautifully! Thank you.

Thank you Julie Mueller, Jennifer Weitzman and your team at JamGD for another beautiful book cover and graphics. Great work!

Big thanks to Rachel Elkind for perfectly capturing my happy mug at the Union Square Farmer's Market in New York City. It was hard work navigating through all of those healthy shoppers, but you did it. I love my headshots!

Thank you to my students and clients who have found the courage to question their medical protocols and start taking on the process of healing their thyroid conditions naturally. Every day, I am inspired and am learning new things from all of your experiences.

Thank you Valerie Feder for giving me many opportunities to share my voice with a much larger audience. And, thank you Lily Feder, just because.

And, of course, a BIG thank you to my hubby, Pablo Garcia, for allowing me to fully express myself, even if, on many occasions, you wished that I wouldn't. Thank you for always reminding me that many of the things I say may *not* be accepted by mainstream society and could possibly rock some boats. Thank you for being a great support system for me as I fully express myself to the world. I love you.

INTRODUCTION

If you ask what I wanted to be when I grew up, my answer is probably one you would never expect. In my imaginary ideal life, I was a rock-and-roll disc jockey spinning the classics. I wanted to be the voice on the radio guiding you through an awesome playlist that touched you to the core and brought you some happiness.

Becoming a thyroid expert and advocate for natural healing was nowhere on my agenda. But, the Universe had other plans for me.

What started out as finding my own path to naturally healing thyroid disease turned into discovering my life's passion: teaching others how to heal using whole foods and natural healing methods.

What I've learned over the past twenty years about healing the thyroid is contained within these pages, and that information is needed now more than ever. Take a look around, and you may realize that almost everyone you meet nowadays has been diagnosed with thyroid disease or they are suffering from its exhausting and often debilitating symptoms.

I was diagnosed in 1996, and at that time, I was informed by doctors that my thyroid condition was incurable. I chose not to accept their "incurable" diagnosis, and by naturally healing my thyroid using the strategies in this book, proved my doctors wrong. Their idea that a disease is incurable is what they had been taught in medical school, but it isn't necessarily the whole truth.

Since healing my condition, I've gone on to share my voice and teach countless others around the world how to heal their thyroid conditions, too. I have seen the results in my own life and the results from clients and students who share their amazing stories with me.

I want you to get ready because it is possible to heal your thyroid naturally. You no longer have to suffer from debilitating symptoms:

- Weight problems
- Hair loss
- Dry skin
- Chronic fatigue
- Depression
- Anxiety
- Infertility
- Muscle and joint pain
- Goiter
- Heart palpitations
- Menstrual irregularities
- Tremors
- Sleep disturbances

Once you understand your thyroid better, you can get to the root cause of your condition, and your symptoms will begin resolving themselves. That's the beauty of natural healing.

The body you are living in is absolutely perfect! I know you may not feel as though it is, but it is.

If you are suffering from symptoms of thyroid disease, it is your body's way of speaking to you and letting you know that something is amiss and needs adjusting. Your thyroid is actually giving you warning signals. The quality of your nutrition, stress levels, immunity, circulation, emotional health, and environment are all factors that need to be assessed and addressed.

Many people begin suffering from symptoms of thyroid disease and get tested to discover that it's either too slow or too fast, or not producing enough of the hormones needed to function properly. The answer in modern medicine is to take some type of thyroid hormone to lessen the symptoms, or to have the thyroid irradiated or removed.

A dear friend had her thyroid removed a few years ago. The doctor assured her that the thyroidectomy would eliminate the symptoms she was experiencing. He was correct. Her symptoms did go away for about six months. But, they came back within one year because she never got to the root cause of the problem.

Why was her thyroid out of balance? What was it trying to tell her about her overall condition and her diet and lifestyle?

The thyroid, as you'll discover in this book, is not the root cause of the problem. Feeling out of balance is just a symptom of a deeper issue, and the thyroid is the communicator that is letting us know.

Taking thyroid hormone or destroying the thyroid is NOT the answer to *healing* a thyroid condition. To properly heal the thyroid, we need to get to the root cause of the symptoms. Is something not quite right with the person's diet? Are essential nutrients missing? Is the person under some type of stress, either emotional or physical? Is the body depleted? What's happening in the physical environment?

Stress, both physical and emotional, includes pregnancy! I know a LOT of women who get diagnosed with thyroid disease when they are pregnant or just after giving birth—there is a reason for that.

The baby takes most of the mother's nutrients to grow, so the mother is left depleted and suffering from chronic fatigue syndrome or adrenal fatigue. For those of you old enough to remember, this used to be called postpartum depression, but I guess that's passé now, and thyroid disease is the latest trend in medical diagnosis.

Other physical stressors include overworking, taking on too much, and not getting enough rest. How many of us actually get sufficient rest? We are a society that is functioning on fumes. If you are constantly on the go with very little down time, it can set the body up for thyroid disease, adrenal fatigue, and many other diseases.

If someone is suffering from an autoimmune thyroid condition like Hashimoto's or Graves', we have to look deeply into the digestive system for clues to healing. The majority of our immune system lives inside there, and we cannot heal until we dive in and see what's going on.

There are many underlying factors in understanding and eventually healing thyroid conditions, and we'll cover them throughout the pages in this book. Western medicine focuses solely on the thyroid, or separate parts of the endocrine system, but looking at the body that way is limited in scope. It's not the whole picture.

Don't get me wrong... Western medicine has an important role in our life, but it's not in *healing* thyroid disease.

Throughout the years, I've met with many other people who have tried to heal their thyroids naturally by changing their diets, but they were unsuccessful. They tried gluten-free, dairy free, vegan, raw foods, paleo, supplements, herbs—you name it! And, they were still suffering from thyroid disease and didn't know why.

I even met with clients who have actually *given* themselves thyroid disease by taking on what they thought was a healthful diet. Unfortunately, what many people have been taught is healthful throughout the past few decades may actually be weakening and destroying the body instead.

Be patient. We'll cover all of these eye-opening topics, one chapter at a time.

Throughout this book, I advise, above all, to be patient and loving with your body as you go through the process of healing. If you want your thyroid to be fixed by the end of the week, you are reading the wrong book.

Another reason some people do not heal their thyroid disease is because they don't look any deeper into their condition. They stay at the surface and focus solely on the physical body. They get their blood checked, monitor their TSH, T3 and T4 levels, and chase their tails around and around and around, focusing on their hormone levels: "My T3 is low." "My TSH is high." " I don't have enough T4." As you'll discover in this book, it's all nonsense!

When I was going through the process of healing, my thyroid jumped from hyper to hypo to Hashimoto's; my hormones were all over the place. If I had intervened with medication at any point during my healing process, I would have stopped my body from finding its balance.

There is so much more to healing the thyroid than just looking at blood work. Human beings are multifaceted creatures with many layers. We are more than just our skin, bones, and blood. We are physical, emotional and spiritual beings. To heal disease, we have to look deeper:

- Where did this disease come from?
- What am I supposed to learn from this condition?
- Why is this happening at this time in my life?

A wise teacher once told me, "All disease comes from spiritual sickness." At the time, I was focused only on food and didn't understand what the heck he was talking about! But, after working with thousands of students and clients, I know he was correct.

There may be a higher purpose for the condition you are suffering from at this time in your life. I want to encourage you to bravely go into those painful places within yourself to discover the truth about your thyroid condition.

I've worked with many clients to help them get beyond their symptoms, discover the root cause of their thyroid condition, and finally heal. I've also worked with people who do NOT heal, and I'll share case studies as we go through this book together. You may begin to see yourself more clearly through someone else's struggle or someone else's success.

Healing is a process that takes time, especially when you're dealing with the endocrine system and the emotional body. These are systems responsible for long-term changes, so again, patience is the key.

I met a woman at a conference where I was the keynote speaker. She had a very large goiter and was suffering from hypothyroidism. She told me she had been trying to naturally heal her thyroid condition for over a decade! That indicates something may not be working with her approach. Although I do emphasize patience, ten years is a long time. I've seen people heal their conditions in three months to three years of taking on this journey.

You, too, can heal your thyroid condition. I'll share with you the information that can help guide you toward success. If you're reading this book you may fall into one of these categories:

- **You have been diagnosed with some type of thyroid disease**
- **You have all the symptoms of thyroid disease but haven't been diagnosed yet**
- **You have thyroid disease and want to get off the medication**
- **You're on medication and still suffering from many of the symptoms**
- **You were recently diagnosed and you are looking for alternative ways to heal**
- **You no longer have a thyroid and want to know what to do for the rest of your beautiful body**
- **You have taken radioactive iodine to destroy the thyroid, but you're still not feeling well**
- **You are working with people with thyroid disease and want to help them to the best of your ability**

If any of that rings true for you, reading this book is exactly where you want to be. The information contained herein can show you how to finally get to the root cause of your thyroid condition, reclaim your health, and start living a happier and healthier life.

One of the greatest things that you will experience from healing your thyroid is confidence in your body's ability to do what it is designed to do. If you can heal your thyroid, you can potentially heal any condition that comes up for you in this lifetime.

My thyroid disease has been a blessing. It has taught me that the power to naturally heal a disease that is inside me is inside every human being on the planet. All it takes is a bit of unconventional courage, an open mind, and some stick-to-itiveness to reclaim your body's innate wisdom and power.

Your thyroid disease could quite possibly be the best thing that has ever happened to you. Trust me, I know it may feel like this is the biggest pain in the neck (pun intended!), but your thyroid is going to teach you so much about yourself and your journey here on the planet.

Are you ready to heal your thyroid condition? If yes, I encourage you to keep reading!

Let me be the voice that guides you, step by step, through a playlist of natural healing methods, so you can discover what it's like to live your life with a happy, healthy thyroid.

CHAPTER 1
From Sickness to Wellness

Prior to my diagnosis of thyroid disease, I spent twenty-eight years being mostly disconnected from my physical, emotional, and spiritual body, and not fully supporting its needs. I didn't know how to care for the flesh, blood, and bones I was living in, and I didn't know what my body needed from me on an intimate level to thrive. In turn, my body couldn't show up for me either; it was breaking down and malfunctioning in subtle, and not so subtle, ways.

At the time of my diagnosis, I was working as an Executive Assistant at MTV networks and had been feeling run down. My two LARGE cups of coffee per day were slowly steeping their way toward three. On top of that, I consumed at least two cans of Diet-Pepsi every day.

You would think that with all that high-octane caffeine stimulating my system, I would have enough energy to make it through the average workday, but I didn't. By one-thirty in the afternoon, my eyes grew irritated and dry, and I couldn't keep them open.

Using a pile of unfiled paperwork as a pillow, I plopped my head down in front of my computer screen to take a fifteen-minute nap. Thankfully, my boss escaped the office every day for long leisurely lunches, so my naps went largely unnoticed.

The odd thing was, even though I was feeling physically exhausted, I had trouble sleeping at night and suffered wild bouts of insomnia. I found relief drinking shots of NyQuil, but it always left me groggy as heck the next day. I felt as though I had a horrible hangover without the benefits of a fun night out on the town with my friends.

I also experienced random moments of uncontrollable anxiety and stress. I would be sitting at my desk typing on the computer, not exerting myself strenuously in any way, and my heart would race uncontrollably. If this has *never* happened to you, imagine the vibration of a machine gun releasing rapid-fire rounds.

Badabadabadabadabadabadabadabadabadabadabah!!! It was nerve-wracking and left me feeling anxious about a potential heart attack at the tender age of twenty-eight!

Chronic fatigue, insomnia, and uncomfortable heart-racing symptoms weren't the only indicators that something was amiss. My immune system was weak, and I suffered from frequent colds and bouts of flu that lasted way too long. Once a respiratory ailment caught hold of me, the coughing and congestion lingered for weeks, and sometimes months. I became the cough-drop queen! I was always slurping on a symptom-soothing candy: cherry mint, honey lemon, original herb, and cooling menthol. They were yummy, but didn't actually help. I constantly cleared my throat of some mysterious congestion that never seemed to fully resolve itself.

For me, the worst part of having a weakened immune system was the unsightly cold sores that made regular appearances on my lips, nose, philtrum (the area between my lips and nose), and chin. It seemed that no area around my mouth was safe from the shameful blistering and scabbing. Oh the horror! I would call out sick from work for a few days until the fiery blister subsided. But, the scab always remained for at least seven to ten days to remind me, and everyone else who glanced in my direction, that I was cursed with the dreaded herpes virus!

Another interesting symptom: I was freezing *all* the time. No matter what I did, I could not warm my body, especially my extremities. My hands felt like carved ice blocks. When I wasn't typing at the computer, I would sit on my hands to warm them. I also remember bundling myself up in sweatshirt, sweat pants, and sweat socks at bedtime, but it didn't help. The cold sensations were coming from inside, not outside, my body.

The symptoms that ultimately brought me to the doctor's office were chronic sore throat, laryngitis, and a swollen neck. My diagnosis arrived wrapped up in a goiter-shaped gift box that said, "Congratulations, you have thyroid disease."

The doctor informed me that my hyperthyroid condition was incurable and recommended I take radioactive iodine to destroy my thyroid and then to take Synthroid (synthetic thyroid hormone) for the rest of my life.

Radioactive iodine was not an option for me. Years earlier, I witnessed the devastating effects of radiation on my mother's body and vowed never to put radioactive *anything* anywhere near me, especially not inside me. You can read about my eye-opening experience with my mother's breast cancer in my first book, *The Whole Truth – How I Naturally Reclaimed My Health and You Can Too!*

I told the doctor I wanted to improve my diet and my lifestyle instead of destroying my thyroid with radiation. She told me my diet had nothing to do with my thyroid and that my condition was "incurable."

The doctor was correct. According to what she learned in medical school, my condition was indeed incurable. Thankfully, I didn't go to medical school, so I had a different perspective. I was willing to give my body the ingredients it needed for a fighting chance to heal.

I left the doctor's office with a focus on healing my body. It was time for me to step up, improve my diet and lifestyle, and learn how to properly care for myself. From the time I was in my early teens, I was obsessed with dieting and the need to be ultra thin like the models in the popular magazines. It's funny that growing up, I was a skinny little kid. I didn't actually start gaining weight until after I went on my first diet at fourteen years old.

For as long as I can remember, I was always on some type of diet, seeking, but never obtaining, weight loss. I was up, I was down, but rarely was I ever happy with my weight. At my plumpest, I was 149 to 153 pounds, which by no means is fat, and may not seem heavy to some folks, except that I'm 5' 4" on a tall day. And, according to the ideal weight charts, I was in the "overweight" range.

As a teenager, I was chubsy-ubsy for sure. I wore sweat pants most of the time, because squeezing my butt into a pair of jeans was downright uncomfortable, and I refused to buy the next size bigger pants.

The weight I gained as a teenage dieter refused to leave my body no matter how often I dieted. Whatever fat I released while dieting always seemed to reattach itself to me... like a bad relationship–which it certainly was! My relationship with food was downright dysfunctional.

I had been on every diet imaginable: Slim Fast, Jenny Craig, Weight Watchers, The Cabbage Soup Diet, Fruit Only Diet, Vegetables Only Diet, Fat-Free Diet, High Carbohydrate Diet, The Grapefruit Diet, and many others. I was always depriving myself of some major food group – carbohydrates, fats, or proteins. I didn't eat sensibly; I just followed the guidelines of the latest weight loss fad.

There were also times that I didn't eat anything at all. I would take Dexatrim over-the-counter diet pills or weight loss pills prescribed by a doctor in Long Island.

When I took those diet pills I would eat NOTHING for days at a time. And, right before my high school prom, I didn't eat anything for an entire week! That's seven days with zero food. Just water and diet pills. Egads!

My crazy dieting behavior created an endless cycle of bodily stress. Plus, I had a love/hate relationship with my bathroom scale. On days that I was one or two pounds lighter, I wanted to get down on my hands and knees and kiss the little white metallic bathroom creature. Yay!

But, on the days that I was heavier or the same weight as the day before, I would start torturing myself, and my body, for failing. I was bulimic for quite a few years. I alternated between throwing up and taking daily laxatives to try to poop my weight down the scale.

The scale ruled my life. Whatever the scale said in the morning would set the mood for my day. If I didn't like the number on the scale, I would think all day long about how "fat" I was or how much weight I needed to lose. It was a constant stressor, and I know today that stress contributes to weight gain and poor health.

On a typical dieting day, I would start with coffee, artificial sweetener, and skim milk. I drank that every morning until I discovered soymilk. I thought soymilk was a better option for me and it became my go-to, guilt-free, creamy liquid. Some days for breakfast, I would have a caffè latte and a whole wheat bagel, dry – with nothing on it but air. Bagels aren't meant to be eaten that way, but I was afraid of cream cheese, butter, or any type of fat. Other mornings, I would scarf down instant oats with maple syrup and a splash of soymilk.

My midmorning snack was fat-free or low-fat cookies or a granola bar, or on a "good" day, an apple. For lunch, I would line up with the rest of the herd at the local salad bar trough and eat a big bowl of raw vegetables with fat-free or low-fat dressing.

Sometimes I would indulge in a slice of pizza with the greasy cheese peeled off and discarded in an orange stained napkin that sat on the side of the table. Occasionally, I would sneak a bite of that fatty cheese, but I always felt guilty afterwards. Damn that cheese! I was convinced that brief moment of enjoyment is what kept me fat!

In the early afternoon, right before my daily nap at my desk, I would pop a handful of Skittles or plain M&M's into my mouth because they didn't have any fat. I would, of course, wash it down with a Diet Pepsi.

A few times per week, I took the elevator down to the frozen yogurt shop in the building to indulge in a guilt-free, nonfat or low-fat frozen yogurt with crumbled peanut butter cups sprinkled on top. Because the peanut butter cup was *deconstructed* the calories must have somehow escaped. Usually, I finished my day with a big sensible salad and a piece of grilled chicken or a tuna fish sandwich with low-fat mayonnaise on whole wheat bread.

At that time, I thought my typical day of eating was healthful compared to most other folks. I mean I wasn't eating fast food like Burger King or McDonalds, and I wasn't sitting down to a big fat T-bone steak with French fries.

I also went to the gym religiously three to four times per week and climbed the StairMaster to nowhere for at least fifty minutes, and sometimes an hour. For the life of me, I couldn't understand why the heck I wasn't shaking those excess pounds off my butt.

The truth is, I was living a dieting nightmare. I was eating mostly high-carbohydrate meals with low-fat foods and copious amounts of salad. Plus, I was exercising really hard even though I was physically exhausted. I know today that all of those behaviors contributed to my weight problem and to my thyroid disease.

When I finally snapped out of that dieting mentality and instead focused on healing my illness, the weight naturally dropped off within about three months. And, I have kept it off for almost two decades with absolutely no fear of it coming back. Clearly, focusing on healing my thyroid disease turned out to be the best diet ever!

It's an amazing feeling to heal the body of an "incurable" condition. It's empowering. It helped me build confidence in my body's ability to do what it is naturally designed to do: function properly.

I've discovered that all you really have to do is give your body what it needs, and it will reach its ideal weight without much effort. By remaining focused on the goal of healing the body instead of the triviality of weight loss, I have learned amazing things about life, health, and well-being. Healing the thyroid is not solely about eating a nourishing diet. Food is only the first step in this journey. The human body needs proper physical nutrition, reduction in stress, and emotional and spiritual healing to become balanced and to properly heal.

The extreme eating and lifestyle of my past may not reflect your story, but I can guarantee you will find an abundance of useful information and clients' stories that you can identify with in the upcoming chapters. As you read through this material, please keep in mind that healing doesn't happen overnight. Healing takes time. I had a client from Texas who was suffering from hypothyroidism. She had a very large goiter, much bigger than mine, plus she was forty pounds overweight and was feeling terribly depressed. Her doctor told her she needed to take medication, but she didn't want to. She said she had seen me on *Top Chef* and was intrigued when I said I healed my thyroid condition naturally. She searched for me on the web and signed up for health coaching.

The first thing we did was get her off all of the processed foods, junk foods, and diet foods she was consuming and drinking on a daily basis, and put her on a whole foods diet. Within thirty days of improving her diet, she lost twelve pounds and was feeling excellent! She was amazed at how quickly her body responded to real food. She went back to the doctor and took another blood test. Her thyroid hormone levels read completely normal. That was the quickest any of my clients had ever normalized their thyroid blood work. Healing the thyroid can take anywhere from three months to three years depending on a person's condition.

Although her thyroid numbers were normal, the downside to this woman's condition was that she still had a very large goiter. The doctor recommended that she take medication, as it was the only way to reduce that goiter. She questioned that because he had also told her that she needed medication to normalize her hormone levels.

I told her to be very patient. I said, "It took time for the goiter to grow and it'll take time for that goiter to reduce. My own goiter took eighteen months to disappear!" Here is a picture of my lovely little goiter.

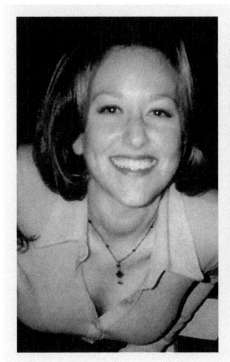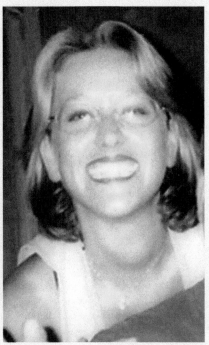

I had another client from upstate New York whose goiter was even bigger than the gal from Texas. It took two years, and a lot of patience, for her goiter to resolve itself. With natural healing, especially with anything that has to do with the endocrine system, patience is the key. One of my favorite quotes by Ralph Waldo Emerson is a great reminder for us:

"Adopt the pace of nature, her secret is patience."

Remember to be patient. Your body can heal when given the right nutrition, love, and self-care. You are going to learn what you need to know to heal your condition, but you need to understand that it's not going to happen overnight.

Many people may feel that being diagnosed with a disease is one of the worst things that could possibly happen to them. My thyroid disease taught me valuable lessons about my body and woke me up to a whole new way of eating and living. Having this disease was truly a blessing that inevitably improved my health and my entire life as well as the health of countless clients.

The first step to healing a thyroid condition is to gain awareness of what may be happening and why. After that there are many steps to healing, and I'm going to share them with you one chapter at a time.

So, before we set the table and sit down to eat a yummy thyroid-nourishing meal, I'm going to teach you the basics about your gorgeous gland, how or why it may not be functioning properly, and what you can do about it.

CHAPTER 2
Thyroid Shmyroid – What the Heck is it Anyway?

Before we can heal the thyroid, we've got to get to know it on an intimate level and understand all of the amazing functions it is responsible for inside your body.

SEE HUMAN ENDOCRINE SYSTEM DIAGRAM ON PAGE 18

The thyroid is a butterfly-shaped gland located just below the center of the neck. It lives on the endocrine system with its brother and sister glands–the hypothalamus, pituitary, pineal, parathyroid, thymus, pancreas, adrenals, and gonads (ovaries and testes).

These endocrine glands secrete hormones that evoke specific responses in cells, tissues, and organs throughout the body. The endocrine system is one of our main communicators, using blood to deliver hormonal messages to the cells, making them more permeable. It's fascinating the way the body communicates with itself without our having to do *anything* except simply exist in the world!

For the purpose of this book, we're focusing mainly on the thyroid, but not solely on the thyroid as Western medicine might do. We're not going to isolate and segregate your thyroid gland as if it is the cause of your disease, because it's not.

Contrary to what we've been told by most medical professionals and mainstream society, the thyroid gland may *not* be responsible for the ailments and discomfort so many people are experiencing.

A malfunctioning thyroid gland is merely a symptom of an *entire* system that is out of balance. For that reason, this book focuses on the entire mind/body system as a whole, rather than just one little piece of it.

The thyroid is where we are starting this journey because that's what got you here. But, the thyroid is probably not where the dysfunction originally began.

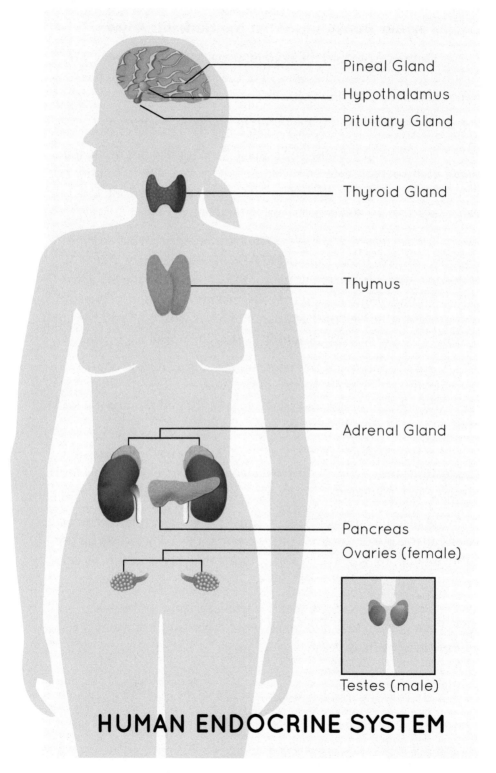

Pineal Gland
Hypothalamus
Pituitary Gland

Thyroid Gland

Thymus

Adrenal Gland

Pancreas
Ovaries (female)

Testes (male)

HUMAN ENDOCRINE SYSTEM

These are some of the common thyroid dysfunctions:

- Hashimoto's thyroiditis or Autoimmune thyroiditis – an autoimmune disease causing inflammation of the thyroid gland, which manifests itself most often as hypothyroidism, but can cause hyperthyroidism as well
- Hypothyroidism – underactive thyroid not producing sufficient thyroid hormone
- Hyperthyroidism – overactive thyroid producing too much thyroid hormone
- Graves' disease – autoimmune disease that can cause hyperthyroidism
- Goiter – enlargement of the thyroid gland that can be caused by either hypo- or hyperthyroidism, or by ingesting too little or too much iodine
- Nodules – benign (noncancerous) lumps on or around the thyroid
- Thyroid cancer – malignant lumps, nodules, cells

"The function of the thyroid gland is to take iodine, found in many foods, combine it with the amino acid tyrosine, and convert it into the thyroid hormones thyroxine (T4) and triodothyronine (T3). Thyroid hormones are then released into the blood stream and transported throughout the body where they control metabolism, which is the conversion of oxygen and calories to energy. Every cell in the body depends upon thyroid hormones for regulation of its metabolism."[1]

The thyroid is responsible for metabolism of oxygen and glucose, and that means it's a pretty darn important gland! But, then again, *all* of the glands in the human body are essential to our optimum functioning. That's why they are there.

What amazes me about modern medical treatment and diagnosis is the focus on the thyroid gland as if it is a solo operator. Keep in mind that the thyroid does NOT work on its own. Remember, it lives on the endocrine system. That means there are many more factors at work supporting, or not supporting, the proper functioning of this gland.

For example, the pituitary and the hypothalamus (glands located in the brain) control the actions of the thyroid. If thyroid hormone levels drop, as in the case of hypothyroidism, the hypothalamus secretes

1   http://www.endocrineweb.com/conditions/thyroid/how-your-thyroid-works

Thyroid Releasing Hormone (TRH) and alerts the pituitary gland to produce Thyroid Stimulating Hormone (TSH).

The thyroid, if receptive, responds to the orders delivered from the brain by producing more or less hormone. If the thyroid is not responding or functioning properly, we need to look at some of the other glands in the body as well. Most certainly, we need to check in with the hypothalamus and pituitary glands because they place the orders for more or less hormone.

If the thyroid is not "receptive" to the orders coming from the brain, that's a key issue we need to understand to help heal this disease. The behavioral problems of our glands' failure to communicate effectively with each other will be covered in the chapters ahead.

The thyroid regulates our metabolism, which is the body's ability to break down food and convert it into energy. Food is fuel for the body, and everyone burns it at a different rate. Some people are quick burners, and some people are slow burners.

Generally, people with hypothyroidism and Hashimoto's are characterized as slow burners, having a tendency to gain weight and having difficulty losing it. On the other hand, people with hyperthyroidism are usually quick burners, as the name suggests ("hyper"!), and can have trouble gaining weight.

Modern medicine treats the thyroid without taking the entire body and mind into consideration. Treatment for hypothyroidism can include using synthetic hormones to unnaturally speed up a sluggish thyroid. This may seem like a good idea, but can be highly detrimental and doesn't get to the root cause, throwing the body even more off balance.

Ask some of the folks who have taken synthetic hormones for hypothyroid conditions for a few years (or just check in with yourself), and see if their symptoms are still present or have gotten worse. Initially, many folks feel better and more energized, but within a few years they often complain of feeling worse... much worse!

They begin noticing that other problems have suspiciously taken root, like adrenal fatigue (chronic exhaustion), osteoporosis, bone fractures, muscle weakness, sleeplessness, irregular heartbeat, breast or reproductive cancer, liver stress and toxicity, hair-loss, and overall poor immunity.

So many clients have complained to me about feeling worse after taking synthetic thyroid hormones that I'm surprised more doctors haven't taken notice of this. It makes me wonder if those clients are speaking up and telling their doctors what they are telling me. Speaking up and sharing your truth, in a gracious and effective way, is part of healing the thyroid on a deeper level.

There have also been recent studies that have indicated thyroid medication can lead to early-onset dementia and Alzheimer's[2], so maybe those clients are simply forgetting to tell their doctors what is going on with their health.

Almost every day, I receive emails from people worried about their TSH (thyroid stimulating hormone) levels, or wondering how to improve their T3 or T4 (thyroid hormones) levels. I always encourage those folks to stop focusing on the hormone levels in the blood tests. Those tests are not accurate in the process of healing thyroid disease. It's called "chasing the numbers," and it doesn't work.

When I was initially diagnosed with my condition of hyperthyroidism and goiter, I was suffering from many of the symptoms of hypothyroidism as well: weight gain, hair loss, brittle nails, dry skin, lethargy, premenstrual syndrome, and bouts of anxiety and depression.

I refused the recommended treatment for my thyroid condition (radioactive iodine and a lifetime of thyroid hormone), and instead, focused on improving my diet and lifestyle. As I altered my diet, my blood work began changing as well. Each time I went for another blood test, my thyroid had shifted into a new form of thyroid disease. First it was hyper, than it was hypo, then it was Hashimoto's thyroiditis.

My thyroid hormone levels were all over the place!

But, my physical body was improving daily, weekly, and monthly. I disregarded the blood tests and the doctor's fears about my condition and listened to my body instead. I've been through many incarnations of this disease. I've also witnessed many clients transform from one condition to the next as their bodies attempted to rebalance themselves. It's truly fascinating!

---

2   http://www.ncbi.nlm.nih.gov/pmc/articles/PMC2820146/

Our food creates our blood, and that blood feeds all of our organs, systems, and glands, including the thyroid gland. It's basic common sense that as you adjust the quality and type of food you are eating, your blood would feed your thyroid new nutrients it may have been lacking before.

If I had focused solely on my blood work, without looking at the BIG picture, and intervened with medication at any time during my healing process, I would have hindered my body's natural healing process.

The body is a self-healing organism. It is perfectly designed, and if we give it what it needs, it can heal itself. Going for periodic blood tests is great—they can show you what may be happening inside your body at any time. Or, they could create a false sense of worry and stress if you get stuck chasing the T3, T4, and TSH numbers in the blood work.

We need to look at the body in a much bigger way. The symptoms of thyroid disease are the body's way of telling us that something is out of balance.

If you want to heal your thyroid condition, it would be wise to focus on getting to the root cause of the disease instead of treating the symptoms and the numbers with medication. When the thyroid is not functioning properly, there may be many underlying reasons for this. You need to start asking yourself questions:

- Am I getting proper nourishment?
- Am I overworked?
- How are my stress levels?
- Am I overeating sugar, stimulants, or carbohydrates (that includes whole grains, beans, and starchy vegetables)?
- Have I neglected good quality protein and fat (vegan diet)?
- Have I neglected good quality carbohydrates (paleo diet)?
- Are my adrenals fatigued?
- Do I have mercury fillings in my teeth? Root canals?
- Am I eating too many refined foods high in iodized salt?
- Am I using chemical sweeteners?
- Do I have digestive problems?
- Am I chewing my food properly?

These are just a few of the many possibilities why the thyroid may be out of balance. NONE of these possibilities can be found on your thyroid blood test.

It's time to focus your attention on getting to the root cause and finally healing your thyroid condition. Whether you have hyperthyroidism, hypothyroidism, Hashimoto's, Graves', nodules, goiter, hyperparathyroidism, hypoparathyroidism, or thyroid cancer, there may be an underlying reason for that condition that you and your doctor are not aware of.

If your thyroid gland is out of balance, we need to do some detective work to discover how and why it got that way in the first place. Otherwise, the underlying problems will persist and continually wreak havoc on your system.

With diet and lifestyle improvements, you can successfully restore thyroid function by treating the underlying causes of the condition. Keep in mind, there may be *many* contributors to thyroid disease, and we are going to cover them in this book. You are going to need to practice patience and understanding while trying to figure your condition out.

Another common treatment for a malfunctioning thyroid is to attack it as an enemy of the body. Radioactive iodine is one way to do this, especially for Graves' disease and hyperthyroid conditions. This therapy was recommended to me when I was first diagnosed. Thankfully, I declined! But over the years, I've seen many clients who have taken the radioactive iodine treatment.

For those of you who do not know what this is, I'll give a brief overview: Radioactive iodine, taken either in pill or liquid form, is absorbed by the thyroid gland. It destroys the thyroid, but supposedly does not harm other tissues in the body.

According to WebMD, "To avoid exposing other people to radioactivity, it is important to follow your doctor's instructions carefully. He or she will instruct you on how far to stay away from people, how long you need to sleep alone, and other ways to stay safe. You will be directed to avoid close contact, kissing, sex, and sharing cups, dishes, or utensils."

There are many other general recommendations for someone who has taken the Radioactive Iodine treatment:

- Flush the toilet twice each time you use it.
- Use separate towels, washcloths, and sheets. Wash these and your personal clothing by themselves and not with other people's laundry.
- Use a special plastic trash bag for all your trash, such as bandages, paper or plastic dishes, menstrual pads, tissues, or paper towels. Talk to your treatment facility to see if they will handle the disposal. Or after eighty days, this bag can be thrown out with your other trash.
- Don't cook for other people. If cooking is necessary, use plastic gloves and throw them away in the special plastic trash bag.
- Wash your dishes in a dishwasher or by hand. If you use disposable dishes, they must be thrown away in the special plastic trash bag.
- You should not breast-feed your baby after you have been treated with radioactive iodine.
- If you plan to travel on the interstate, you may set off radiation detectors. Most police and transportation workers are aware of medical radiation, but it may be a good idea to carry some paperwork from your doctor.

Many of these precautions are to insure that you do NOT expose other people to radioactivity. I've had clients who have taken the radioactive iodine tell me that their doctor told them not to touch another human being or pet for five full days after taking this treatment.

Here's some wise advice: if someone, no matter what his or her credentials, ever tells you to "drink this liquid or take this pill, and then do NOT touch any other living creature for five days," run as fast as you can in the opposite direction.

Trust me on this… think twice before you drink the Kool Aid. For those of you too young to remember this catchphrase, it refers to the mass suicide at Jonestown, Guyana, where the followers of the Reverend Jim Jones trusted him blindly. Over 900 cult members died drinking the poisoned liquid he dished out to them.

Another extremely radical thyroid treatment is thyroidectomy, the removal of the entire thyroid or pieces of it. It seems it is becoming more "normal" than ever to assault the body rather than support it.

Do you remember how popular lobotomies were in the 1940s and 1950s? Some medical professionals were performing them to help cure headaches, mental illness, and criminal behavior. We know today that treating the brain by cutting out portions of it is not a smart idea. Always question the medical authorities, especially when they want to cut out pieces of your body.

Trends happen all the time in food, fashion, media, and medicine. Thyroidectomies are the latest surgical trend presented by mainstream medicine as a solution for hyperthyroidism, goiter, and thyroid cancer. It may be an overly aggressive approach and an entirely unnecessary procedure.

When I was growing up in the 1970s, tonsillectomies were all the rage. At seven years old, I had a traumatic accident and needed eleven stitches to close a gaping wound across the bridge of my nose. After surgery, I remember sitting in the hospital bed with white gauze taped across my face, listening to the doctor advising my mom to let them remove my tonsils. He asked me to open my mouth so they could get a look inside. Then he showed her my irritated, enlarged tonsils, and handed me a mirror so I could see them too. They looked like big, red poisonous mushroom caps sprouting from the inside of my throat.

He asked if I had frequent colds and throat infections. Both my mom and I told him my throat was constantly swollen, and that I lost my voice often and was frequently sick. He suggested that, while I was in the hospital, he could quickly remove my tonsils and reassured us I wouldn't be as sick in the future.

The doctor was condemning my tonsils for creating the many maladies I was experiencing in my young life. In truth, many of the food choices I reached out for had contributed to my poor health. At the age of seven, I was already a full-blown sugar junkie, constantly compromising my immune system with sweet, nutrient-depleting substances. Pop Tarts, Captain Crunch, and candy were my staples. My irritated tonsils were loudly advising me to "STOP!"

Thankfully, my mom declined that unnecessary tonsillectomy, and I left the hospital intact. Removing an organ, gland, or body part is a costly procedure, and it doesn't "cure" any disease. The body part itself may not be the cause of the dysfunction. Hearts do not cause heart attacks, brains do not cause strokes, breasts do not cause cancer, tonsils do not cause tonsillitis, and thyroids do not cause thyroid disease.

Here's a little fact that makes perfect sense. "In the United States, the number of tonsillectomies has declined significantly and progressively since the 1970s."[3] It was an overly aggressive procedure that didn't cure anything. We know today that it is NOT wise to remove the tonsils because they play an integral part in immunity and stopping future infections.[4]

In the same way, removing or destroying the thyroid will NOT cure a thyroid condition. The thyroid is not the cause of thyroid disease. Something else is going on internally that needs to be addressed before doing any sort of radical medical procedure.

According to ancient wisdom, the thyroid is our great communicator. It is warning us that we are out of balance on many levels and need to get realigned. We need to listen to what this beautiful little gland has to say, not silence her forever.

If you are being advised to have your thyroid removed, irradiated, or destroyed in some way, I would suggest you take a moment to rethink that advice. I am encouraging you NOT to fall into the trap of destroying your thyroid gland. Once the thyroid is removed or obliterated, there is no turning back.

If you are reading this book and you are missing your thyroid, or pieces of it, or have taken radioactive iodine, it's time to be gentle and loving with yourself. It is essential that you support your adrenal glands, the rest of your endocrine system, and your body as a whole. Send your body love, and assure it that you are the caretaker and you are learning as you go. Just keep moving forward from this point on with your remaining organs, glands, and systems intact. Your body will love you for taking a stand and protecting it.

In upcoming chapters, we'll talk about "protection" and how it relates to the thyroid. For now, let's check out another couple of glands that have a deeper connection to thyroid disease, and most people don't even know it.

3   http://www.entnet.org/content/tonsillectomy-facts-us-ent-doctors
4   http://www.livescience.com/34476-what-are-tonsils.html

CHAPTER 3
Stress and The Adrenal Connection to Thyroid

You would be surprised how many thyroid conditions naturally resolve once the adrenals have been properly nourished and supported. It's amazing!

The adrenals live on the endocrine system and they produce estrogen, progesterone, cortisol, cortisone, adrenaline, epinephrine, norepinephrine, and dopamine. They are located on top of your kidneys, and they are integral to your immune system and to the functioning of your thyroid.

The adrenals are considered the batteries of the human body. They are responsible for our energy levels and endurance, and can keep the body going and going and going, like that little Energizer Bunny from the television commercials in the '80s.

If that reference is too old for you, try this one: when you purchase a toy for the kiddies, it simply won't run without the batteries—and, neither will we.

The adrenals also help us recover from disease. It's imperative that while we're healing the thyroid, we fully support our adrenals. If our internal batteries (adrenals) run low, we won't be able to heal any thyroid conditions, or healing can take an extra long time.

Our adrenals also help us cope with everyday stress and survival. We are all exposed to stress, no matter who we are or where we live. There is no guaranteed way to avoid the stresses of life, but there are many ways to deal with them to make life more manageable and enjoyable.

Please take note that many of the symptoms of thyroid disease are also symptoms of adrenal fatigue:

- Brain fog
- Lightheadedness
- Dizziness
- Low blood pressure
- Poor immunity

- Exhaustion
- Hair loss
- Depression and anxiety
- Insomnia
- Decreased sex drive

The human body is perfectly designed and filled with an internal wisdom many of us cannot comprehend. The body will always try to achieve balance, and when the adrenals are exhausted, it will naturally start conserving energy for survival. The body is protecting itself. This can naturally slow the body down into a hypothyroid state.

Underlying factors can contribute to adrenal fatigue and disrupt thyroid function:

- Nutritional deficiencies
- Recurring illnesses
- Chronic infections
- Constantly "going and going and going" without adequate rest
- Sleep deprivation
- High sugar/carbohydrate intake
- Excessive caffeine and stimulants
- Overexercising
- High stress (both physical and emotional)

Number one on our list is nutritional deficiencies. That's pretty easy to understand. If the physical body isn't getting what it needs on a cellular level, the system starts breaking down.

I've had many female clients complain of being diagnosed with hypothyroidism either during their pregnancy or after childbirth, especially if they are breastfeeding. The baby takes *most* of the mother's deep nutrition.

If the mother is not getting enough of the nutrients she needs, she will become deficient. Once she becomes deficient, the thyroid will naturally slow the body down.

The baby, dare I say, is a parasite! It takes from the host (mother) for its survival. The organism hosting this growing parasite is the mother's physical body. Once again, the body is wise and does not want to expire before its time, so it naturally slows all processes. The body is brilliant!

Some nutrient-dense foods I highly recommend for pregnant women, new moms, or anyone suffering from adrenal fatigue and other deficiencies are bone stock and organ meats, especially liver, from both land and water animals. Pregnant women in indigenous cultures around the world were given liver and other highly nutritious foods to eat while pregnant.[5] Scientifically, we know that animal liver contains the highest concentrations of protein, vitamin B12, vitamin A, Vitamin D, and heme iron, which is more absorbable than the nonheme iron found in plants. When a pregnant woman goes to the OB-GYN, she is given a prenatal vitamin that contains all of these nutrients, with an emphasis on iron that helps build the blood and feed the fetus.

Many people suffering from thyroid disease can also suffer from anemia and deficiencies of vitamins B12 and D. A nutrient-dense pregnancy diet that helps deeply nourish and support the kidneys and adrenals can aid the thyroid as well. Keep in mind that you do NOT need to eat for two. You just need to eat more nutrient-dense foods. I certainly don't want you gaining weight on a thyroid-healing protocol, unless of course, you need to.

This doesn't mean you need to eat a LOT of liver or other organ meats. You don't. Liver is so nutrient dense that you only need to eat a little bit if you are suffering from deficiencies. In the recipe chapter, I will teach you delicious ways to prepare various types of food, including liver, to support the body's need for deep nutrition.

I've had many students and clients turn their noses up at the mere thought of eating liver. But, after they've tasted liver that has been prepared properly and tastes delicious, they change their minds and their picky palates.

I also highly recommend bone stock for anyone suffering from nutritional deficiencies. Bone stock is a magical elixir. In many cultures around the world, women were given bone stock after giving birth to help them refuel and energize their bodies. Bone stock was also traditionally given to anyone suffering from wasting diseases, which prevent nutrients from being absorbed. Bone stock is an easily absorbable liquid form of minerals and collagen and is GREAT for healing and supporting the digestive system.

People suffering from digestive disorders like irritable bowel syndrome, Crohn's, colitis, or any of the autoimmune thyroid conditions like Hashimoto's and Graves' disease should be consuming bone stock on a regular basis to help support and heal their intestines. Over 70 percent of the immune system lives in the gut and needs to be nourished properly to help heal those pesky autoimmune thyroid conditions.

---

5   http://www.westonaprice.org/health-topics/sacred-foods-for-exceptionally-healthy-babies-and-parents-too/

According to Sally Fallon, founding president of the Weston A. Price Foundation, there's an African proverb that reminds us that "a good stock will resurrect the dead." So, if you're feeling like you're *dying* and have little or no energy, bone stock would be a great choice.

I had a client, Martha, who was suffering from thyroid disease and goiter. She was a small business owner and worked long days and nights. She didn't have a large enough support team, so she did most of the work herself. Martha told me that for two years prior to her diagnosis, she was feeling completely drained of energy, but the doctors couldn't find anything wrong with her. She said, "Even after eight or ten hours of sleep, I am still groggy and feeling wiped out." Her doctor had recommended antidepressants.

Her symptoms spoke volumes! She was suffering from an underlying adrenal fatigue, and that led to her being diagnosed with a thyroid condition years later. I encouraged her to take some much-needed breaks during the day (including a nap) and to incorporate a daily helping of bone stock into her diet. Within two weeks she started feeling more energized. She called me and told me she wanted to get her thyroid tested again to see if it had healed.

I told her to relax and be patient. Even though she was feeling better, it could take a few months, or a few years, for her thyroid hormone levels to test normal. And, it would certainly take time for her bulging goiter to reduce in size.

The beauty of bone stock is that you need to make a batch only once or twice per month to fulfill your bodily needs. You don't need to eat or drink stock all the time. In the warm weather, especially, it can be too rich, heavy, and dense.

If you are currently suffering from osteoporosis, digestive disorders, or adrenal fatigue, you may want to have stock on a daily basis, even during the warm summer season. You'll know when it's time to stop. You'll feel a sense of fullness and deep satisfaction. In the coming chapters, I'll cover how to know what your body needs on a deeper level.

Osteoporosis, by the way, can take up to seven years to heal, so you have to be very, very patient with that condition. Many of the thyroid medications contribute to both osteoporosis and renal failure.

It's one of the reasons I recommend getting off the meds as soon as you can, if you can. The only reason to take thyroid hormone is IF you no longer have a thyroid or have had the radioactive iodine treatment.

Now, back to bone stock. It is very easy to prepare, and I've shared some simple recipes with you in this book. For those of you who don't want to cook bone stock, you could purchase it online, or go to your local farmers market and check in with the meat and livestock farmers. Ask if they are making stock with the bones from their animals. There's actually a pretty BIG market for homemade stocks right now, and for good reason. They are needed in the world! Human beings, generally, may be suffering from being overweight; paradoxically, even many who are overweight are seriously undernourished.

One of the main factors in our rampant nutritional deficiencies could be our highly refined, high sugar, high carbohydrate diet. That is how I personally discovered adrenal fatigue.

There was a time, in my early thirties, when I was practicing a vegan diet and eating only grains, beans, vegetables, fruits, nuts, and seeds. A vegan diet can be highly beneficial for people suffering from diseases of *excess*, but it may not be good for all people.

All of the vegetable-based foods I was eating were high in whole grain carbohydrates, vegetable starches, and beans. When I would eat a plate filled with grains, beans, and vegetables, which seemed like a pretty balanced natural foods diet, it was contributing to blood sugar spikes and malabsorption of nutrients in my body. Eating rice and beans and vegetables without any saturated fat and/or animal protein to help slow its absorption would bring my blood sugar up, and then crash it down again. I was constantly hungry and found myself grazing the cupboards all day long!

Plus, I wasn't fully absorbing the fat-soluble nutrients because the vegan way of eating was too low in fat and protein for my body. Had I been vegetarian instead of vegan and eating eggs and dairy with my meals, that may have helped.

I've seen similar types of nutrient deficiencies and blood sugar imbalances in many of my vegan clients. Over time, a high-carb way of eating can exhaust the adrenals and the pancreas in some people.

My adrenals and pancreas could not keep processing that large dose of carbohydrates at every meal three times per day plus snacks. My digestive system was stressed out, and I crashed! My blood pressure was 80/50. My immune system kept tanking. I was dizzy and felt faint when I stood up. It was awful!

I thought I was eating the "most healthful" diet in the world but I was actually missing some essential nutrients. Adding animal protein and saturated fat back into my diet helped to increase my blood pressure, and I felt more balanced and started absorbing nutrients on a deeper level. I felt the difference all the way down into my bones.

What I've learned from both my personal experience and from my clients' experiences with a vegan diet has convinced me NOT to recommend a vegan diet for healing the adrenals or the thyroid. It doesn't mean that you cannot have vegan meals. Just don't have them three times a day every day for many years. That can be problematic and lead to adrenal fatigue, candida overgrowth, and bone loss too.

Except for the overwhelming exhaustion and other symptoms mentioned at the beginning of this chapter, you may not even suspect you have adrenal fatigue. Many medical professionals find this condition only at the tail end in the form of Addison's disease. Addison's is when your adrenals have called it quits! They cannot put out any more hormones. They stop working and take a much-needed vacation.

Barbara was a client who had been on thyroid medications for over ten years before being diagnosed with Addison's. Her underlying condition began with adrenal fatigue, but she was erroneously diagnosed with hypothyroidism and was put on a synthetic hormone to speed up her thyroid.

The truth is... her body wanted to S...L...O...W down, and that's what it was doing: slowing down. With Addison's disease, the body can take a very long time to heal. She began feeling better soon after altering her diet and lifestyle; within three months, she was feeling more functional.

If your body is slowing down due to underlying adrenal fatigue, thank your thyroid for saving your life. Say, "Thank you thyroid – you're a wise teacher. I need to de-stress, I need to slow down, and I certainly need to learn to relax."

I want to emphasize that stress is a normal and healthful part of life. It is *excess* stress that harms us and depletes our adrenal energy.

For example, if there is a lion in my vicinity, and it's hungry, and it's looking at me, I absolutely, 100 percent, want my stress hormones to kick into high gear and send energy to my muscles and extremities, so I can run as fast as possible to save my life! After I reach a safe distance, I need my other stress hormones, as well as my parasympathetic nervous system, to kick in and help my body come back to a state of normalcy and relaxation. I'll need to calm down.

Stress is essential for our survival. The problem with modern stress is that it is *chronic stress,* which completely exhausts the body's reserves and causes us to break down. Our bodies CANNOT keep up the daily demand for stress hormones.

Here's a common scenario of how *excess* stress works in our everyday world: A working mom wakes up and has to rush to get the kids ready for school, and then get ready for work. Then she has to get to the office, but she's stuck in traffic. Once she finally arrives at the office, she has deadlines that have to be met, and there are other people in the office who are bothering the crap out of her! She can't get her work done. She sits at her desk and rushes through lunch, barely chewing her food. Another pile of work gets plopped onto her desk, and she has to stay late. Then she has to get home to make dinner, eat, and listen to the kids fighting with each other. By 8:00 p.m., she is lucky to be alive and may be wishing that she would've gotten eaten by a lion instead.

How many of you can identify with that scenario? I know it may be a bit extreme, but that's the way some of us have our lives set up. We're constantly going and going and going, and we're simply not designed to handle that pace. We are not battery-operated bunnies.

Overwork is a stressor that depletes energy. Too much work without adequate rest is not healthy. Unfortunately, this is what *most* modern folks are doing every day. Work, work, work, work, work, and then work some more!

I always remind clients that no matter how hard they are working, they have to remember to take their lunch breaks, set boundaries around work commitments, and leave the office on time. There is more to life than just work. We have to have balance in our lives, otherwise we'll exhaust ourselves.

And, if you're doing work that you do *not* enjoy, that can make you feel even more depleted. You will spend your days grinding away at a job, just for the money, and not receiving joy from it. Talk about exhausting, ugh!

If you have consistent days filled with overwork and chronic stress without adequate rest and relaxation, there will nothing left for your body to give. When you're going through a life that looks and feels completely stressed, your thyroid will slow down. It simply can't keep up with that kind of craziness. Unless, of course, you have super adrenals, then your body will be hyped up without slowing down, as in hyperthyroidism and Graves'.

Many of my clients diagnosed with hyperthyroidism and Graves' have very high stress levels, both physical and emotional, and they do NOT know how to relax. We have to discover ways to de-stress, otherwise we're going to ruin our health.

Modern thyroid medications speed up a slow thyroid so it can keep up with the crazy stressed-out lifestyles we've created. This is one of the main reasons many people taking medication for hypothyroidism can begin feeling even more exhausted after a few years. The body cannot keep that kind of speedy pace. It just can't.

In the case of hyperthyroidism, those folks are given medications to slow their thyroids or stop them from working entirely. But, that never gets to the underlying stress either.

As we continue moving forward, I'll teach you easy relaxation techniques, and how to deal with the people in your life who may be stressing you out: kids, boss, partner, or the person who accidentally crossed your path at the wrong time while you were rushing to work at a job you don't enjoy.

Until we get to the relaxation techniques in this book, I just want you to make the mental note to slow down. Be patient...relax. Take a deep breath, or two or three, and calm your system down. Whether you have hypo, hyper, Hashimoto's, Graves', goiter, or thyroid cancer, it's time to relax.

I know it's difficult to slow down because we think we have to keep up with the unnatural pace that society has created. I'm going to suggest that you begin questioning that pace. You don't have to do everything. You do have to do *something*, but you do not have to do *everything*.

The next stressor we're talking about is OVERexercising! Yes, there is such a thing. Exercise is essential to keep the body functioning properly, but we need to have a balance of many different types of exercises to be truly healthy.

Another client of mine, Kathleen, was a high level marketing executive. She loved her job, but it was stressful at times. She also ran four or five mornings a week before getting into the office, and did a spin class twice per week.

You would think with that amount of exercising, she would have no problem with her weight, but she did. She had hypothyroidism and could not lose that nagging twelve pounds that had been weighing her down for over a decade. She was frustrated that she could implement the best marketing strategies to win clients, but when it came to losing weight she was struggling.

We altered her diet, and I encouraged her to consider cutting back on her strenuous exercising to only two times per week running or spinning, and to incorporate daily walking and gentle Hatha Yoga classes into her routine as well.

Kathleen was extremely hesitant. Her greatest fear was that if she stopped working out so hard she would blow up like a balloon, But, when she finally moved beyond that fear and let her body relax, she lost ten pounds the first month. She was shocked! She thought she had to starve herself and exercise her brains out to lose weight, but that wasn't true. She just needed a more balanced approach to the way she was exercising.

A young male student who attended one of my thyroid health cooking classes was running over seventy miles per week. Holy cow— that's a lot of running! He was suffering from hypothyroidism, and he couldn't sleep at night. Sleeplessness can actually be an indicator of adrenal fatigue. His doctor told him to "stop running!" I agreed with the doc's wise assessment. This student was running himself right into adrenal fatigue.

Keep in mind that running won't necessarily contribute to thyroid disease, but if you add nutritional deficiencies and high stress to an overexercising routine, your body may be headed for a breakdown, or, I should say, a slowdown. If you are overexercising and not doing enough rejuvenating and restorative activities as well, you could drain your body's deep energy reserves.

For all of you ladies out there who are still getting your menstrual cycle every month: STOP exercising when you get your period, especially on the first and second day of your cycle. Exercising while you are bleeding is exhausting!

Think about it this way – you are shedding the uterine lining, which is like having an internal operation every month. That takes a physical toll on the body. You have to rest during that *special* time of the month, otherwise you may damage your reproductive system and your reproductive capacity as well.

On the first day of your period, it's time to rest. If you want, do some simple stretching or deep breathing exercises, but no hardcore exercising. Relax, take a walk, chill out, and get a massage.

If you need a reminder, think back to what you learned when you were a child in school. If there is a *period* at the end of a sentence that means STOP! It's not a comma, where you would pause or take a breath and keep going. It's a period. STOP!

Exercise is imperative to good health, so keep exercising, but know when to run and when to rest. I would highly recommend adding some rejuvenating practices like QiGong, Tai Chi, yoga, and meditation into your exercise routine. It could do wonders for your health. We'll cover that in the upcoming chapters.

Something else that drains our batteries is chronic infections, and that can include root canals and other infected teeth. Any time your body's immunity is being forced to work overtime, it drains energy.

Over the years I've heard from many clients who have had work done on their teeth and who say that they just didn't feel right afterwards. Some of them tell me they suffered from tinnitus (ringing in the ears), dizzy spells, vertigo, and recurring sinus infections after having root canals.

Most of these people intuitively felt something was happening inside that particular tooth, or underneath a cap, or in a root canal. If you "feel" something uncomfortable in your body, no matter what it is, it's time for you to begin trusting your instincts and intuition. That's part of connecting to your thyroid gland and to the *truth* of what is happening inside your body.

Any chronic conditions, like cancer and candida overgrowth, that you may be suffering from can also drain the health of the adrenals. You can find health supportive information about cancer and candida on my website **www.AndreaBeaman.com**.

It's time to go a little bit deeper and look at emotional and mental stress and how that can affect the health of our adrenals and thyroid. Mental stress can bring disease faster than anything!

Mental stress is thoughts, and thoughts travel very quickly—faster than the speed of light.

I've got a great example for you. After the attacks on the World Trade Center on September 11, 2001, people in New York City were pretty shaken up. I remember that every day on my block on the Upper East Side of Manhattan, there was another moving truck. It was wild to see so many people exiting the city so quickly, but it was understandable. People were scared.

I had a dear friend who was suffering from the mental stress of the *possibility* of another attack on the city. She was having a hard time functioning. She could barely get to work in the morning, and she was afraid of everything because her thoughts of another possible terrorist attack were consuming her.

She was so stressed out that her gorgeous curly brown hair was falling out in clumps. High stress and prolonged stress lead to adrenal fatigue, which can cause hair to fall out.

One day, I met my frazzled curly-haired friend downtown for lunch. She told me she couldn't travel on the subway anymore.

She said, "What if there's another attack on the city and I'm on the subway… I won't be able to get out… I might suffocate down there… I could get trampled by other people… I can't be underground when it happens again… I just can't do it. I don't want to die underground!"

I told her that I understood what she was going through, and that she was correct. There certainly could be another attack in New York. We live in a city that is a high profile target. The truth is, the next time the *entire* city could be destroyed. Even though New York City is considered one of the biggest cities in the world, it's relatively small in size.

Her eyes grew wide with fear.

"But," I said, "before you freak out, I want you to follow my line of thinking here. We're sitting at this restaurant, and there is a glass of water on the table. What if I knock over that glass, and it falls onto the floor, shatters, and goes into my foot? I'll have to go to the hospital to get the glass removed. But, I don't have any health insurance, so it may cost me a few thousand dollars. I don't have a few thousand dollars laying around. So I won't get treated and then my foot can become gangrenous, and I'll have to get it cut off, and then I'll have one foot, and I won't be able to work anymore! I won't be able to stand in the kitchen and cook. I won't be able to pay my rent, and I'll get kicked out of my apartment, and I'll be homeless!!"

And, she said, "Oh my God, Bea, that's awful!"

I said, "Yes, oh my God is right! But... what is the truth here?"

She blinked her big brown eyes a couple of times and stared at me.

I said, "The truth is... the glass is still on the table. None of that stuff I was thinking about has actually happened. Yes, there's a possibility of it happening—just like anything can happen at any time. But, if I live in the world of potential catastrophes, I can't possibly live happily and healthfully in the world right now."

The kind of emotional stress my friend was suffering from, the stress that was making her hair fall out in clumps, was in her mind. She was stuck up there, spinning around and around and around, because she lost sight of the truth. The truth will always help you find your way, and it can set you free from anxiety.

It takes practice to get out of your head and get into the world. Especially after a traumatic event.

It seems many of us are either projecting in the future, fretting and worrying about what could possibly happen, or we're stuck in the past, depressed about what has already happened, unable to move forward from it.

Not being present is not a healthful way to be in the world, and it can suck the life out of you. I'm going to cover how to get present to help you find the truth and de-stress. For now, just remember to relax and breathe.

What is happening right now at this very moment? You are reading a book and learning information about healing your thyroid condition. Keep moving forward at the pace you are going and try not to get ahead of yourself. You'll get all the information you need at exactly the right time that you need it.

Any time we are under prolonged mental or emotional stress, it can drain our adrenals and energy reserves and that can affect the thyroid. I've met with clients who were diagnosed with hypothyroidism or adrenal fatigue soon after the death of a loved one. Death is a BIG stressor! I know it's not an easy subject, but death is a part of life.

Birth and death are happening all the time, and we can't have one without the other. When we lose someone we love, a partner, a pet, a family member, or a friend, the trauma and stress of that death takes a toll on us. The grieving process kicks in, and when that happens, bodily functions may naturally slow down and become depressed.

This is normal.

What's *not* normal is when we can't rebound from the loss of a loved one. If we can't recover from the death of a loved one, our own desire to be alive wanes, and that can zap our adrenal and our kidney energies.

Our adrenals sit on top of the kidneys, and according to traditional Chinese medicine, the kidneys store our life force, or our "*jing*" essence. If we do not have the desire or the will to continue on after the death of a loved one, our own life force becomes depleted. The kidneys feel it, the adrenals feel it, and the entire body feels it as well. Your kidneys are responsible for your will and your ability to move forward in the world.

When people are diagnosed with thyroid disease shortly after the death of a loved one, it is not a coincidence. It is very likely the result of the emotional stress taking a toll on the memory center in the brain and on the adrenals, which can affect the thyroid.

It happens all the time.

I'm going to suggest to anyone suffering from the loss of a loved one that you allow yourself to fully grieve that loss. Feel it all the way down into your bones. Then release it. Then feel it again, and release it again. Thoughts and memories will come up over and over again, and you just have to cry it out and let it go. The feeling of loss is going to come in waves. When it does, let those painful waves wash over you, and cry. It's normal and healthful to experience our emotions.

We are perfectly designed creatures, and we are prepared for our emotions to move through us. Our little tear ducts keep the eyes moistened and clean, as well as help us shed emotions through crying.

That dearly departed soul whom you loved had an impact on your life and touched your heart. Cry when you need to, and release any unexpressed feelings. Then take a deep breath, and come on back to the world.

Death is a part of life, and we simply can't have life without it. It may help you to think about this quote by Kahlil Gibran, "When you are sorrowful look again in your heart, and you shall see that in truth you are weeping for that which has been your delight." It's one of my favorite quotes and helps me get through the tough times when I miss the folks who have exited this life before me.

Weep tears of joy when thinking about the people who have impacted your life. They are no longer here in the flesh, but I'm sure they would want you to be enjoying life because YOU are still here.

I didn't say healing the thyroid was going to be easy, but I did say it was possible. There may be some tough stuff you have to go through, but you can get through it.

There are many other things that can drain our energy, compromise our adrenals, and lead to thyroid disease. In the following chapter, you'll discover some of the environmental factors that can contribute to thyroid disease.

Before you turn the page, take a moment or two to breathe and relax. Whenever you're ready, let's keep going.

Chapter 4
What on Earth is Going On?

After a nuclear disaster, large populations of people can suffer some form of thyroid disease or thyroid cancer. Examples of these disasters would be the explosion at the Chernobyl Nuclear Power Plant in Ukraine (1986), and more recently, the earthquake and tsunami that destroyed the nuclear power plants along the coast of Japan (2011).

Two decades after the explosion, the World Health Organization stated the Chernobyl nuclear disaster will cause 50,000 new cases of thyroid cancer among young people living in the areas most affected by the fallout. And, due to the high levels of radioactive iodine that were released into the air, soil, and water, many others will develop hypothyroidism.[6]

From the Fukishima disaster, studies are showing a rise in thyroid cancer among young children in Japan.[7] There has also been a 28 percent increase in thyroid problems in babies born *after* the Fukishima disaster in cities on the Pacific Ocean in Alaska, Hawaii, California, Oregon, and Washington.[8]

In America, we had the Three Mile Island (TMI) accident in Middletown, Pennsylvania, in 1979. According to the United States Nuclear Regulatory Commission, the small radioactive releases had no detectable health effects on plant workers or the public.[9] But, the United States National Library of Medicine, after a 30-year follow-up, told a different story. "Thyroid cancer incidence since the TMI accident was greater than expected in the counties analyzed when compared to local and national population growth. This supports a link to chronic low-level radiation exposure and thyroid cancer development."[10]

Beyond these large-scale nuclear disasters, there are many everyday exposures that can compromise the health of the thyroid, too. Some of the seemingly most benign things we are exposed to on a regular basis can disrupt the thyroid's ability to function properly. We've accepted them as "progress," but they may not be as harmless as they appear.

6   http://thyroid.about.com/cs/nuclearexposure/a/chernob.htmc
http://www.who.int/ionizing_radiation/chernobyl/backgrounder/en/
7   http://www.theguardian.com/world/2014/mar/09/fukushima-children-debate-thyroid-cancer-japan-disaster-nuclear-radiation
8   http://www.washingtonsblog.com/2013/04/study-almost-one-third-of-babies-born-after-fukushima-in-alaska-california-hawaii-oregon-and-washington-have-thyroid-problems.html
9   http://www.nrc.gov/reading-rm/doc-collections/fact-sheets/3mile-isle.html
10   http://www.ncbi.nlm.nih.gov/pubmed/23371046

Cell phones, computers, iPads, televisions, microwave ovens, and other electrical appliances all emit electromagnetic frequencies and low levels of nonionizing radiation. Although neither have been *directly* connected with DNA damage or cancer, they affect our cells in other ways.

The industries selling these products have suggested the amount of negative energy given off by these technologies is below the government's exposure standard. For the sake of your health, please question the government's standards.

Up until 2005, I did NOT have a cell phone. My friends and family would complain, "When are you getting a cell phone? Join the modern world already!" But I was a holdout. I had no desire to be reached while I was taking a relaxing stroll through Central Park or chilling out with a cup of herbal tea at a coffee shop. Chill-out time is something we all need, but many of us do not get.

As fate would have it, in 2005, I was picked by NBC/Bravo for a new show that was casting chefs. It was *Top Chef*. My audition for the show was held in California, and I live in New York City. It was a very hush-hush audition, and everything about it was secretive. I didn't know where I was going or what was going to happen when I got there. The only thing I did know was that I would be picked up at LAX airport and taken for testing.

My brother-in-law said, "You cannot take off to California and not be able to contact your family. Enough is enough! You need a cell phone!"

I finally gave in. And, within a few hours I was connected. That's how quickly things happen in our world.

I arrived in California and was sequestered in a hotel room for seventy-two hours while being subjected to the various forms of testing: psychiatric tests, cooking tests, and an overall evaluation by the producers. During that seventy-two hour period, I had the opportunity to use my new cell phone.

The first day, while talking to my sister for approximately thirty minutes, I noticed the side of my face where I held the phone felt hot. I switched the phone to the opposite side and that side heated up as well. I had to keep switching back and forth from side to side. It was uncomfortable.

The second day, during the call home to my family, I started developing a slight pain in my jaw and on the side of my neck. It was a weird achy pain. I thought maybe it was from the way I was holding my head while talking on the phone. So I made sure to keep my head in a straight, upright position and not tilt to one side or the other.

By day three of using my new cell phone for approximately thirty minutes, I felt constriction in my neck and a definite pain was developing in my thyroid. It was intense. I was feeling the effects of holding that cell phone up to my face near my neck. It was clearly having an effect on my thyroid. The thyroid gland is damaged by radiation. The cell phone emits low levels of nonionizing radiation.

When I got home from California, I made a mental note to use the cell phone infrequently and for emergencies only. Plus, I got a set of ear buds (earphones), so I would NOT hold that thing anywhere near my face and neck.

An interesting thing happened two years after my initial cell phone experience. I met a man who worked for one of the largest phone companies in the United States, and we got to talking about, of all things, cellular phones. He told me that he never *ever* puts a cell phone up to his face. He also said that the cell phone tower repair contractors are warned not to spend more than one hour inside the cell phone tower. One hour!

I don't know if what he was telling me was true. I don't have any facts to back up *his* statement about the workers' contracts with the cell phone company, but I cannot deny my own experience using a cell phone. I certainly couldn't imagine being near or ON a cell phone tower that constantly emits much higher radiation frequencies. What effect *does* that have on the contractors working on those towers?

Recently, I read an interesting article that said working on a cell phone tower is one of the most lethal jobs in the United States with between one and four casualties per month.[11] Those casualties are due to "falling." I can't help but wonder *why* these workers are falling in such large numbers (much higher than loggers, who also work at tall heights). Is something happening to their brains and nervous systems while they are up there near the cell phone tower? Radiofrequency and electromagnetic frequencies (EMFs) are directly responsible for the heating effect that happens to human tissue, the same heating effect I

---

11   http://www.heraldtribune.com/article/20070921/NEWS/709210477?p=1&tc=pg

felt on my face when using a cell phone. Maybe working on the towers is literally frying the workers' brains and disorienting them. For the sake of their health, and their lives, they may need to wear protective radiation suits to ensure their safety.

Back here, down on the ground, people talk on cell phones for *hours* at a time. Most of the people I know have even gotten rid of their landlines and use their cell phones for all of their communications. Some folks even use those Bluetooth thingies that concentrate low-level radiation and EMFs directly onto the side of the head. Eeek!

The National Cancer Institute says, "Cell phones emit radiofrequency energy, a form of nonionizing electromagnetic radiation, which can be absorbed by tissues closest to where the phone is held. A recent study showed that when people used a cell phone for 50 minutes, brain tissues on that same side of the head metabolized more glucose than did tissues on the opposite side of the brain."[12]

The researchers noted that the results are *preliminary*, and possible health outcomes on brain cells are still "unknown." The National Cancer Institute says "more research is needed."

Really? That's enough research for me to NOT put a cell phone to my head, but for those who are not yet convinced, keep reading.

A recent study in the Journal of Experimental Biology shows that EMF exposure impacts both the structure and function of the thyroid. For example, animals exposed to cell phone radiation produce lower levels of thyroid hormone, a marker of hypothyroidism.[13]

Keep in mind that modern medicine uses radioactive iodine to STOP the thyroid from functioning. Cell phones emit low levels of nonionizing radiation. My suggestion for you is NOT to put a cell phone anywhere near your thyroid!

Use the speaker option or get some darn earphones. I know those earphones are a pain in the butt because they *always* get tangled, and they are constantly breaking, but who cares? This is your health.

Beyond cell phones, we are exposed to computer technology every day, sometimes all day long. If you are sitting in front of a computer screen, a tablet, or an electronic book reader right now, look at where

---

12   http://www.cancer.gov/cancertopics/factsheet/Risk/cellphones
13   http://www.annlouise.com/blog/2013/01/08/is-your-cell-phone-zapping-your-thyroid/

that screen is facing. We sit with the computer technology directly in line with our face, chest, neck, and thyroid. Again, this electronic equipment is emitting low levels of nonionizing radiation and electromagnetic frequencies.

Not only that, if you are looking at a computer screen at night, and this includes your cell phone, you are disrupting the body's natural circadian rhythms. The circadian rhythm is the twenty-four-hour cycle in the physiological process of all living beings, and it is affected by light. It is responsible for determining our sleeping and waking patterns and is directly linked to our brain wave activity, hormone production, and cell regeneration.[14]

When you look at your computer, cell phone, or any other electronic gadget, you are receiving focused light directly into your eyes. That light is transmitted to your pineal gland, affecting your body's natural circadian rhythm. This disturbance can disrupt the nervous and endocrine systems and can keep you up at night, tossing and turning, preventing your getting a good night's sleep and derailing your functioning efficiently the next day. "The (circadian rhythm system) creates a biological night and a biological day so that physiological, and behavioral activities best suited for nighttime, such as rest, memory processing, cellular repair and brain development, take place at night, and those best suited for daytime, such as alertness, and availability of glucose, take place during the day. The prolonged disruption of the circadian synchrony leads to an array of disorders, including insomnias, impaired glucose tolerance and obesity, and decreased life expectancy."[15]

One of the main concerns with man-made electromagnetic fields has been whether the risk of childhood cancers, such as leukemia and brain tumors, has increased because of them. Studies have shown an increase in leukemia in children whose mothers were exposed to high levels of magnetic fields, but, according to these experts, more studies need to be done.[16]

I understand that the experts need more research and studies, but I don't actually need their evidence to tell me that sitting in front of a computer screen all day has an effect on the physical and emotional body.

---

14   http://www.sciencedaily.com/articles/c/circadian_rhythm.htm
15   http://www.patient.co.uk/doctor/pineal-gland-and-circadian-rhythms
16   http://www.cancer.gov/cancertopics/factsheet/Risk/magnetic-fields

When I sit in front of my computer for too long without taking a break, I begin feeling physically drained. Eventually, that physical drain can lead to depression and poor immunity. Mind you, I am in tune with my physical body and can feel when my energy dips. And, it certainly does dip from prolonged computer exposure.

Even though the experts say there is no *conclusive* evidence about cancer specifically, I know that sitting in front of a computer screen is doing something else to the physical body. From an energetic perspective, the body is protecting itself from the electromagnetic frequencies and radiation it is being exposed to, and that can drain the body's physical energy.

Plus, take a look at your computer or cell phone, and you'll notice that it is either plugged into an energy source or it's running on batteries that need to be recharged. Those technologies simply won't run unless they are fully charged or plugged in. The human body needs to be plugged in and recharged as well. Our bodies recharge with proper sleep, sunshine, great quality food and water, and meditation (prayer, spiritual practice), plus exercises like *QiGong* and yoga that can harness the energy that is running the entire universe. According to ancient teachings, there is *Qi* (pronounced chee), or life force, and we have access to it through ancient exercises. I will share with you how to access that energy as you continue moving forward reading this book.

I know many of you, because of the work you do, have to sit in front of a computer all day or for most of the day. It would be wise to get up every hour or two and take a stretch break, or go for a quick walk around the office (or home), and grab a glass of water. I would also highly suggest putting a plant, a small feng shui water fountain, or some rocks beside your computer. Many elements from our natural environment contain negative ions that can help neutralize *some* of the nonionizing and electromagnetic frequencies we are exposed to daily.

Exposing your physical body to the natural environment can also help rebalance and heal the body. Living in New York City (or any busy city) is a far cry from a *natural environment*, but there are still many trees and beautiful parks and beaches that city folks have access to. I use those little blissful places as often as possible to help recharge my batteries. And I always suggest that clients and students do the same, no matter where they are living. I tell them to get the heck outside, away from all the darn technology, and give their bodies a much-needed break so they can recharge, too.

If you are in the process of trying to heal a thyroid condition, or any other bodily ailment, please minimize the amount of time spent on the computer, cell phone, and all of your other electronic equipment. Go out and take a hike! Your body will love you for it.

In addition to the nonionizing radiation and EMF's, we are exposed to something called ionizing radiation as well. Ionizing radiation is *directly* linked to cancer, including thyroid cancer. These specific radiation rays, which cause cells to mutate, can be found in x-rays, including dental x-rays, diagnostic medical x-rays, CT scans, and bone scans.[17] Radiation therapy, which uses radiation as a cancer treatment, can also create secondary cancers and leukemia.[18] Some of you may have experienced some of these secondary cancers already, especially if you've had radiation of the thyroid to treat cancer.

When I was a kid, I remember going to the dentist, and lying in the chair to get work done on my teeth. The dentist or dental assistant would heave a heavy fifteen-pound vest on top of my chest to protect me from the ionizing radiation being emitted from the machines used to take dental x-rays. But my head and neck were still dangerously exposed.

The dentist or the dental assistant would actually leave the room, press a button from a distance, and take x-rays of my teeth. It was very smart of them to leave the room so they wouldn't be directly exposed to those ionizing radiation rays.

One of the editors of this book, Sheilah, added that when she goes to the orthopedist, the technicians put a vest on her and go behind a screen. She said, "The technicians also wear little buttons that show how much radiation they are exposed to." Sheilah said, "I would like to wear one of those buttons!" It's funny—they should really give those buttons to the patients who are being directly exposed to the radiation.

Let's take a look at a technology that is supposed to save us time in the kitchen: microwave ovens. Almost every household in America has one of these modern cooking tools. I understand they are convenient and cook things very quickly, but they are not as harmless as they may seem.

The microwave cooks food by vibrating the water molecules inside the food at very high frequencies, creating extreme friction and heat. During that process, the water molecules are completely denatured,

17   http://www.medicinenet.com/script/main/art.asp?articlekey=47820
18   http://www.cancer.org/acs/groups/cid/documents/webcontent/002043-pdf.pdf

and your food retains that frenetic-type energy. Many studies around the world elaborate on the carcinogenic effects of cooking or heating food in the microwave.[19] But, beyond the studies about microwaves making food carcinogenic, let's get back to the denatured/destroyed water molecules. Your physical body is made up of over 70 percent water. I would be VERY cautious about eating any food that contains water molecules that have been destroyed by the vibrations of a microwave oven.

Always remember that everything you eat is going to become your body on a cellular level. You are what you eat. If the water molecules in your food have been obliterated with frenetic energy, that energy is going to have an effect on your physical/energetic/ vibrational body as well. Your brain, nervous system, and every other cell in your body are going to feel that explosive vibration. Dr. Masaru Emoto discovered that water molecules have energy and structure. His groundbreaking research gained worldwide acclaim after his experiments proved that the quality of our water is deeply connected to our consciousness.[20]

Trust me. Cook your food over a flame the way it has been done for centuries. And, use the microwave only to heat your socks if your feet are cold during the winter.

Next up... some environmental mishaps that could be damaging your thyroid and your overall health.

---

19   http://www.globalhealingcenter.com/health-hazards-to-know-about/microwave-ovens-the-proven-dangers
20   http://www.masaru-emoto.net/english/emoto.html

CHAPTER 5
Environmental Mishaps and Endocrine Disruptors

There are many elements in our environment that have compromised not only the ecosystem but our endocrine system as well. These are called endocrine disruptors. "Endocrine disruptors are chemicals that may interfere with the body's endocrine system and produce adverse developmental, reproductive, neurological, and immune effects in both humans and wildlife. A wide range of substances, both natural and man-made, are thought to cause endocrine disruption, including pharmaceuticals, dioxin and dioxin-like compounds, polychlorinated biphenyls, DDT and other pesticides, and plasticizers such as bisphenol A."[21]

The first batch of endocrine disruptors we're going to talk about comes from our daily food. I cannot emphasize enough the importance of choosing organically grown food or food that is grown without the use of pesticides, herbicides, and fungicides. I wrote about this topic in my earlier books, *The Whole Truth Eating and Recipe Guide* and *Health is Wealth*. Many of the chemicals sprayed onto produce to promote growth and destroy bugs are the very same compounds that destroy our bodies as well.

According to the National Resources Defense Council, many plant and animal species are showing signs of ill health due to exposure to endocrine-disrupting chemicals. For example, fish in the Great Lakes, which are contaminated with polychlorinated biphenyls (PCBs) and other man-made chemicals, have numerous reproductive problems as well as abnormal swelling of the thyroid gland.[22]

We erroneously believe we are separate from our environment, but we are not. What happens to the animals, plants, bugs, and birds happens to us too. Many humans are experiencing problems similar to those of the fish in the Great Lakes.

Here are some interesting facts about a couple of pesticides in particular and about how the government's regulatory system works: Methyl bromide is associated with central nervous system and respiratory system failure in humans as well as having severe deleterious effects on the lungs, eyes, and skin.[23] Methyl bromide has been sprayed on our food supply for decades and is currently being phased out, thanks to the Montreal Protocol of 1987 on Ozone Depleting Substances.[24]

21   http://www.niehs.nih.gov/health/topics/agents/endocrine/
22   http://www.nrdc.org/health/effects/qendoc.asp
23   http://www.epa.gov/ozone/mbr/qa.html
24   http://www.epa.gov/ozone/mbr/qa.html

Hey wait a minute... 1987? As I'm writing this book, it's 2015! That meeting in Montreal was twenty-eight years ago! I understand we are in the process of *phasing this dangerous fumigant out*, but does it really take twenty-eight years? Gosh, our government and the people who are protecting the environment move awfully slowly. Maybe they're suffering from hypothyroidism?

It seems the modern replacement version of that fumigant, methyl iodide, is not much better than its predecessor. In 2010, methyl iodide was directly linked to thyroid tumors, neurological damage, and miscarriages.[25] The EPA assured Americans that they carefully evaluated the risks of methyl iodide and approved it, but with highly restrictive provisions governing its use[26]:

- Shovelers, tractor drivers, and other employees of companies applying the fumigant must wear respirators
- Farmworkers and other farm employees cannot enter the fields for five days after methyl iodide is applied

Really? Everyone applying this fumigant must wear *respirators* and cannot enter the fields for *five days* after? And then I am going to put that food that has been doused with this dangerous fumigant inside my body? Get the heck out of here! Dear EPA, you must be coo coo for Cocoa Puffs or just plain crazy.

If you are one of those folks who think pesticides and fumigants are easily washed off of fruits and vegetables, think again. The plants use soil, water, and air to grow—all of which contain those dangerous chemicals. That means the levels of pesticide and fumigant residue is just as high on the inside of the plant as on the outside. Those are the facts.

The introduction and approval of this dangerous chemical, and others, into the human food supply tells me exactly what I need to know about the EPA and the government's regulatory system. They are not necessarily concerned with the health and well-being of the people.

Please listen carefully because I am about to impart some valuable advice: when it comes to your *health*, do NOT rely on the government to protect you. Always remember that the government is a business, designed to make a profit, and that comes at an expense. You and I are that expense.

---

25   http://www.huffingtonpost.com/2010/06/07/methyl-iodide-controversy_n_602904.html
26   http://www.epa.gov/pesticides/factsheets/iodomethane_fs.htm

The bottom line is clear: chemicals are designed to kill bugs, and they certainly do their job. The difference between human beings and bugs is that we are bigger. It may take longer, but those same chemicals designed to kill the bugs will eventually kill us too.

Buy clean. Buy naturally raised. Or grow your own. Get those hazardous chemicals out of your daily food and out of your beautiful body.

Let's move on to the next endocrine disruptor: Phthalates. The "p" and the first "h" are silent, so it's pronounced "THAHlates." These difficult-to-pronounce little chemicals are also called plasticizers; they are used to make plastic products. Phthalates are in *everything!* From plastic food containers, plastic packaging, sous-vide bags, water bottles, shampoos, soaps, and other personal products—they are ubiquitous. As fate would have it, they have been directly linked with thyroid disease, birth defects, and reproductive and developmental disorders.[27] [28]

One of the keys to keeping phthalates to a minimum is to NOT heat plastic EVER! Heat causes those plasticizers to be released into the food or liquid you are consuming. A plastic water bottle that has been out in the sun or left in your car during a hot summer day will leach plasticizers into the liquid.

Many people are in the habit of putting plastic containers into the microwave to reheat food. This is a really bad idea! If you are home, take the time to reheat food on the stovetop or in the oven. It doesn't take that much time—maybe five to seven minutes. And, if you want to enjoy warm food when you go to the office, purchase an old-fashioned thermos. There are many different sizes and styles to fit your needs.

The next endocrine disruptor is called bisphenol A, or BPA. This is the plastic coating found in many varieties of commercially canned food. The BPA in food and beverages accounts for the majority of our exposure to this hazardous substance. BPA leaches into our food from canned foods, food storage containers, water bottles, and baby bottles too.

The amount of BPA leaching from bottles or food storage containers into our food depends largely on the temperature of the food or liquid that is put into them. To minimize your exposure, do not put *hot* ingredients into any soft plastic containers. And, once again, do NOT microwave any plastic containers. EVER! Let your food cool down before

---

27   http://www.medscape.com/viewarticle/751199
28   http://health.westchestergov.com/bisphenol-a-and-phthalates

putting it into a storage bag or container. You can safely freeze foods in plastic storage containers; just do not *heat* food in them.

When I was growing up in the 1970s, both my parents worked two jobs to support our large family of five kids, two uncles, three dogs, two cats, a few gerbils, 10 rabbits, a couple of snakes, and a turtle. When it came to food, we kids were on our own; we often relied on fast food and frozen food.

I remember a line of frozen Chinese food products that we loved! There was Chicken Chow Mein, Shrimp with Chinese Vegetables, and Beef with Peppers and Onions. It was all cooked, vacuum packed, and frozen into little plastic baggies. All we had do was bring a pot of water up to boil, and drop the frozen plastic bag into the boiling water for about seven to ten minutes. When it was finished, we would simply cut open the bag, and voila—dinner was served!

I would NEVER do that today, especially knowing about BPA and phthalates. That frozen food technology and those types of cooking methods are still available today, but they are no longer just for frozen food.

There is a hot new trend that many chefs are using in restaurants called *sous vide* cooking. It's basically a low-temperature boiling machine. You would place your seasoned proteins into a plastic bag, vacuum seal it, and then drop it into the water for a specific period of time. It perfectly cooks your proteins every time! It's an amazing technology, right? Well… not really.

I was at a chef's conference in 2006 when I first saw that machine. I watched the famous chefs dropping plastic bags into the hot water, and all I kept thinking was, "You have got to be kidding me! Ugh, I eat at their restaurants!"

It's all the rage; many chefs at some of the greatest restaurants around the world are using this new cooking technology. Many home cooks are using it as well. *Sous vide* cooking is a big hit amongst the paleo crowd because of the amount of meat they consume.

When you eat a paleo diet, the amount of animal proteins you are eating on a daily basis is increased; it's basically a meat and vegetable diet. If you burn those meat proteins while cooking them on the grill, in a frying pan, or in the oven, that meat can become carcinogenic. The burning of meat proteins creates heterocyclic amines (HCAs) and polycyclic aromatic hydrocarbons (PAHs). They are chemicals that form when muscle meat is cooked using high temperatures, like grilling over an open flame.[29]

A generally healthy body can handle a small amount of HCA and PAH, so please understand that you can still enjoy the occasional BBQ and grilled meats. But, if you are eating meat three times per day, every day, and damaging those proteins at each meal, that may be excessive and can overload your body with carcinogenic waste.

I've worked with many clients who have taken on a paleo diet and were suffering from thyroid conditions like hypothyroidism, and didn't understand why. Their bodies may not have been getting enough of the glucose needed to support the energy of their cells. We'll cover that information in the food chapter.

The good thing about learning all of this information is that it gives you a *great* reason to eat more home-cooked meals and to eat out in restaurants less frequently. When you cook at home, you know exactly what ingredients are being used and how they are being prepared.

I'm NOT telling you NOT to eat out! I personally *love* going to great restaurants and being served awesome meals cooked by someone else. I'm just informing you of what's going on in the world of food and cooking, so you can become aware of it. Awareness is the first step to healing any condition. Once you are aware, you can make the best choices as often as possible for the sake of healing your thyroid.

Next up on our list of endocrine disruptors is dioxin. It's found mostly in the soil and comes from waste incineration, paper and wood bleaching, and in the production of herbicides. "Dioxin has been demonstrated to disrupt hormone signaling, reduce fertility, interfere with embryo development, and cause spontaneous miscarriage in humans."[30]

A good rule of thumb would be to steer clear of products that have been bleached. This can be difficult for most folks because we like things that look white. The color white is associated with cleanliness and purity.

For the men reading this book, I'm going to apologize in advance for the graphic details I'm about to share with the ladies.

---

29   http://www.cancer.gov/cancertopics/factsheet/Risk/cooked-meats
30   http://www.ncbi.nlm.nih.gov/pubmed/20083559

Tampons: DO NOT put these inside your vagina! Most tampons are bleached. "Swedish studies have shown a link between tampons containing dioxin, and other chlorine by-products, and an increased risk of cancers of the female reproductive tract (especially the uterus, ovaries and bladder). What makes these toxic residues even more disturbing, is that they come in direct contact with some of the most absorbent tissue in a woman's body. According to a doctor at New York University Medical Center, almost anything placed on this tissue, including dioxin, gets absorbed into the body."[31]

There are a few brands of tampons that are not bleached, and you can usually find these in a health food store or natural market. I would suggest using pads most often, or some other sanitary device. And, if you absolutely must use a tampon, make sure you do NOT leave it inside you for long periods of time.

Okay, let's get out of the vagina and back into the environment and onto atrazine. This is an herbicide used on crops and weeds. It has been linked with cardiovascular problems and infertility. Unfortunately, even if you have been buying organic food that has not been doused in pesticides, you may still be getting high doses of atrazine because it has been found in the drinking water. The major source of atrazine in drinking water is runoff from herbicide used on row crops.[32]

Perchlorate is next on our list of endocrine disruptors. "Perchlorate is both a naturally occurring and man-made chemical that is used to produce rocket fuel, fireworks, flares, and explosives. Perchlorate can also be present in bleach and in some fertilizers. Perchlorate may have adverse health effects because scientific research indicates that this contaminant can disrupt the thyroid's ability to produce hormones needed for normal growth and development."[33]

Perchlorate, like atrazine, has also been found in troubling amounts in the drinking water, the groundwater, and the soil. It is directly linked to anemia and thyroid disease, and it disrupts the brain development of fetuses and children. "Children of women with hypothyroidism and high levels of perchlorate during pregnancy have a significantly greater likelihood of having a low IQ."[34]

31 http://www.thebody.com/content/art497.html
32 http://water.epa.gov/drink/contaminants/basicinformation/atrazine.cfm
33 http://water.epa.gov/drink/contaminants/unregulated/perchlorate.cfm
34 http://www.medscape.com/viewarticle/812943

One of the main problems with perchlorate is that it competes with iodine in the body, and, as we know, iodine is essential for thyroid hormone production, a healthy fetal brain, and neurological development. "While iodine is known to be essential for neurological development in the fetus, a recent study published in *The Lancet* was the first to demonstrate that even mild iodine deficiency in utero is associated with lower IQ and reading ability in children."[35]

Unfortunately, because perchlorate has been found in our water supply, it has also been found in most of the produce, including organic, because the farmers are watering the crops with it. If you are getting adequate amounts of iodine in your diet, you won't have to worry *as much* about perchlorate in the water supply. Of course, it would be ideal if we did not have this chemical, or any other chemical, in our water supply. But, we're not living an ideal world. We are living in the world we have created for ourselves, and that means it can be a wee bit toxic. Don't worry! I'll provide you with plenty of iodine-rich recipes to help counteract some of the toxic problems we've created.

The next endocrine disruptor is arsenic. Believe it or not, arsenic in trace amounts can actually be healthful for the body. It occurs naturally in the soil and water. Some studies have shown that arsenic has been beneficial in the treatments of some cancers, like leukemia.[36]

Chronic exposure to arsenic is where the trouble arises. It has been linked to higher rates of many different type of cancers including lung, bladder, liver, prostate, and skin. Arsenic has been given to livestock to help promote growth; it's also used as rat poison, pesticide, and fertilizer.[37]

Unfortunately, plants easily absorb arsenic from the soil. You could actually get chronic exposure to arsenic from eating leafy plants, fruits, and grains that are grown in arsenic-contaminated soil. Arsenic has also been found in higher concentrations in fruit and vegetable juices.

For those of you who have experienced juicing, you know that it takes much more produce to make a fruit or vegetable juice than it does to eat the food in its whole form. That means if you are juicing your fruits and vegetables, you may be getting more arsenic than if you were eating those fruits and vegetables in their entirety. You could eat two or

35   http://www.medscape.com/viewarticle/812943
36   http://www.innovationanthology.com/programs.php?id=144
37   http://theoncologist.alphamedpress.org/content/6/suppl_2/29.full

three whole carrots, but it would take six to eight carrots (or more) to make a glass of juice. This is a good reason to do less juicing. It doesn't mean you can't have fresh fruit or vegetable juice, it just means to have it less often. Eat a whole apple instead of drinking a glass of apple juice. Enjoy some sautéed greens instead of juicing your greens.

There's one more place high concentrations of arsenic have been found. I'll give you one guess, and I'll bet you get it right. As with most of the endocrine disruptors that are in our environment, arsenic has also been found in our water supply. Eek!

This list of endocrine disruptors in our water certainly gives us good reason to filter our water, or at least to have it tested. Always remember to add minerals back into your water if you filter it, otherwise you may become mineral deficient. I know it's not ideal to be adding minerals back into our water, but sometimes you have to do what you have to do, especially when it comes to healing. Pick up a liquid mineral supplement at your local health food store, and follow the instructions on the label.

The ideal is that we have access to fresh spring water or to an underground aquifer, but most of us don't. We have to make do with what we have in the polluted environment we have created.

It's interesting to me that some underdeveloped countries around the world don't have access to clean drinking water, and in industrialized countries we are poisoning our own drinking water with toxic chemicals. We are shortsighted when it comes to our health and well-being and to the health of the planet that sustains our existence.

I remember attending an inspirational event presented by a group called the International Council of the Thirteen Indigenous Grandmothers. If you ever have a chance to listen to these wise elders speak, do it. These are grandmothers from indigenous tribes around the world including Alaska, North America, South America, Central America, Africa, and Asia.

The grandmother from North America, who was about eighty years old, told the audience a story about what her great-grandfather said to her when she was just a little girl. She said, "Great-grandfather took me for a walk. He pointed to the river and to the lake. He told me that there was going to come a time in my life when I was going to have to *know* my food and *know* my water. He said that the days of eating freely from the earth as your ancestors did are coming to an end."

That time has come. We are living it right now.

Many of the things we have done to the earth and to the water, I believe, were originally done unintentionally. As we created more and more industries and dumped our toxic waste into the water supply, we did not realize the horrible ramifications of our actions until the rivers actually caught fire.[38] The infamous Cuyahoga River fire of 1969 sparked a wake-up call to what we were doing to our environment. It wasn't the first time that river, or other rivers in America, caught fire, but it did catch the attention of *Time* and the entire world and alerted us that we had to make efforts to clean up our mess. Today, we are still cleaning up our toxic mess.

There is one known endocrine disruptor that is actually *intentionally* added to our water supply. "For many years now, controversy has raged over whether fluoride should be added to drinking water. As early as 1961, as recorded in the *Congressional Record*, fluoride was exposed as a lethal poison in our nation's water supply."[39] Why the heck is it still in our water? I know the government is slow as molasses when it comes to making changes, but fifty–four years? Really? By the time they get around to taking this poison out of our water supply we could all be suffering from some type of disease, like let's say… hypothyroidism.

"Up until the 1970s, scientists in Europe prescribed fluoride to reduce the basal metabolism rate in patients with an overactive thyroid gland. One published clinical study from this period reported that doses of just two to three milligrams of fluoride—a dose that many, if not most, Americans now receive on a regular basis—were sufficient to reduce thyroid activity in hyperthyroid patients."[40]

More and more information is bubbling up about fluoride and the fluoridation of our water supply. Recent studies have concluded that fluoride alters endocrine function, especially in the thyroid.[41] Independent research by scientists not associated with dental trade

---

38   http://clevelandhistorical.org/items/show/63#.U-TcF1ZcL4g
39   Prescription for Nutritional Healing by Phyllis A. Balch, CNC, Avery Publishing 2006, p46
40   http://articles.mercola.com/sites/articles/archive/2011/08/13/fluoride-and-thyroid-dysfunction.aspx?e_cid=20110813_DNL_art_1
41   http://www.fluoridealert.org/fluoride-dangers/health/thyroid/index.aspx

organizations has found that fluoride [42] [43]

- Is a neurotoxin that accumulates in the brain and lowers IQ;
- Causes cancer;
- Leads to increased hip fractures, skeletal and dental fluorosis, and osteoarthritis;
- Causes birth defects and perinatal deaths;
- Impairs immunity;
- Does NOT provide cavity-protecting effects;
- Suppresses thyroid function;
- Is banned in China, Austria, Belgium, Finland, Germany, Denmark, Norway, Sweden, The Netherlands, Hungary, and Japan.

Why would other countries ban water fluoridation? Maybe they know something we don't. For the sake of your thyroid, all you really need to know is that fluoride is a *"lethal poison,"* and because so many people are so heavily exposed (it's in our drinking water and toothpaste, for gosh sake!), our need for iodine is vastly increased.

There are five halogens (nonmetallic elements found in the periodic table): Iodine, bromine, fluorine, chlorine, and astatine, all of which use the same uptake receptors in the body. Chlorine and fluorine can compete with iodine, blocking iodine receptors in the thyroid gland. Both of those substances are added into our water supply.

Use a water filter that removes fluoride. And, don't brush your teeth with "cavity-fighting" fluoride-based toothpaste. There are many other toothpaste brands, sans fluoride, that can clean your teeth without damaging your thyroid.

Have you got a swimming pool in your backyard? Both chlorine and bromine (two of the halogens that block iodine) are used as disinfectants to keep the water clean and sanitary. Our skin is porous. That means, whatever body of water you are swimming in, you will absorb minute traces of the chemicals through your skin.

---

42   http://www.holisticmed.com/fluoride/
43   http://www.fluoridation.com/c-country.htm

The Swimming Science Journal further explains that[44]

- Exercising competitive swimmers absorb toxic levels of chlorine products;
- Training two or more times a day will not allow the toxins to be completely cleared from the body;
- Children have less developed immune and defense systems, and therefore absorb greater amounts of toxins than older swimmers;
- Dental enamel can be eroded in hyperchlorinated pools;
- Greater toxin absorption occurs through the skin than through breathing;
- Exposure to swimming pool water increases the likelihood of asthma and some cancers.

When you bought your backyard swimming pool, your kids and the neighbors' kids were probably really excited. But truthfully, they and you should not be swimming in highly chlorinated water on a regular basis, especially if you have a thyroid condition.

Here's something you can do: get your waterlogged butt out of the toxic pool, take a hike on a mountain trail with the kiddies, and go jump in a lake. You'd get some exercise and it may be better for your health. Plus, it could be much more fun. If you can't make it to the mountains, grab a blanket and an umbrella, pack a lunch, and head to the beach. Both of those bodies of water may be better for your health than swimming in an ultrasanitized pool that can burn your eyes out of your head!

I clearly remember my eyes burning, itching, and becoming bright red from swimming in chlorinated pools as a kid. Keep in mind that those chemicals are designed to destroy bacteria that can grow in the water. Destroying those bacteria is a good thing, especially in a stagnant body of water like a swimming pool that can become a breeding ground for dangerous bacteria, mosquito larvae, and parasites. But, if nothing can survive in a "clean" swimming pool, not even a frog, you shouldn't be submerging your body in it on a regular basis.

---

44   http://coachsci.sdsu.edu/swimming/chlorine/asthma.htm

The element bromine competes for the same receptors in your body that are used to capture iodine. Bromine can be found in a number of places in our everyday world: [45]

- Pesticides like methyl bromide
- Baked goods and flour products that contain potassium bromate or bromated flour
- Soft drinks, in the form of brominated vegetables oils (BVO)
- Medications in inhalers and nasal sprays or for ulcers and anesthesia
- Fire retardants used in fabrics, carpets, upholstery, and mattresses
- Bromine-based hot tub and swimming pool treatments
- Some toothpastes and mouthwashes
- Hair dyes, deodorants, cosmetics and other beauty products (benzalkonium bromide)

Overexposure to bromine can displace iodine and lead to increased risk for breast, reproductive cancer, and thyroid cancers. In 1990, the United Kingdom banned bromate in bread, and in 1994, Canada did too.

Here's one more environmental toxin I'll share with you, and then we've got to move on; otherwise you're going to want to pack up and move to another planet! This one is not necessarily man-made; this one comes from nature, and it's called mold.

A student in one of my online classes complained of a persistent cough. She said she had been to the doctors and had taken a bunch of tests, but they could not find anything wrong with her.

I asked if she had mold in her apartment. She told me that she had to clean her bathroom and her kitchen every two or three days because the mold grew so quickly in her apartment. Keep in mind that mold can grow in bathrooms, kitchens, and basements because these areas have a tendency to be moist and damp. Having to clean mold every two days means there is an excessive amount of mold spores in the air. There must have been mold in the walls of her apartment or under her floorboards. My advice for that young lady was to move out!

---

45   http://www.huffingtonpost.com/dr-mercola/thyroid-health_b_472953.html

People with weak immunity or adrenal fatigue need to be very cautious about exposure to mold. "If you have a weakened immune system, you may be at higher risk for getting a mold infection. These infections can lead to being hospitalized, or even dying."[46] I'm also going to suggest that even if you have a strong immune system, you don't want to be exposed to mold on a regular basis because it can eventually wear your immunity down.

Many foods also contain molds that can be toxic to our *internal* environment, but we'll talk about those in the food section. For now, please reduce your exposure to mold, pesticides, fumigants, bromine, chlorine, fluorine, and other halogens.

Here's how:

- Eat organic, clean, naturally raised foods, or grow your own
- Avoid fluoridated water
- Avoid soda—this is a no brainer for healing ANY disease
- Get out of the man-made swimming pool, and get into the ocean
- Use natural hair and skin products and cosmetics that are mostly chemical free
- Avoid mold and the dark dank places where it can grow (don't spend too much time in the basement!)

I know this chapter gave you a lot of information to digest, and, trust me, there is more to come. For healing, take every factor that could possibly contribute to your thyroid disease into consideration. It's not just *one* thing that disrupts or damages the thyroid; it could be a multitude of factors.

Try not to overwhelm yourself by feeling that you need to do everything at once. You don't! Just understand that you're moving in the right direction, and you'll get to exactly where you need to go one step at a time.

Remain open to learning and using the information in this book, and be courageous. Always remember that as long as you are alive and breathing, you can improve and/or heal your condition.

---

46   http://www.cdc.gov/cancer/preventinfections/mold.htm

CHAPTER 6
Your Internal Environment and Thyroid Health

In previous chapters, we discussed factors in the external environment that could be damaging your thyroid. Now we're diving a little deeper into our internal environment to see how that can affect the thyroid gland as well.

We're starting with food, but not necessarily with "what" you eat. This has to do with "how" you are eating it. Many thyroid conditions, like Hashimoto's and Graves' diseases, can stem from digestive disorders. Both Hashimoto's and Graves' are autoimmune conditions that can lead to hypothyroidism and hyperthyroidism.

Over 70 percent of our immune system lives in our gut. If the gut is out of balance, immunity can be compromised. We have to heal any underlying digestive problems to successfully treat many thyroid conditions.

The simplest, yet often overlooked, factors contributing to most digestive disorders today are a lack of chewing and *not* connecting to our senses. The face and its sense organs (eyes, ears, nose, and mouth) are the entryways into the inner workings of the body. Through our senses, we connect with what we are eating, how we are eating it, and how it can affect us. Food enters us; it can either nourish us or harm us. Even some of the most "healthful" foods can be dangerous, as you'll discover in another chapter. The face is the first line of defense when it comes to recognizing whether a specific food is good for you.

Our eyes are directly connected to our brain through the optic nerve. Depending on what we are looking at, we can either set our body up for the beginning stages of digestion or we can shut it down.

If we are eyeing a table filled with delicious food, our brain sends a message to the body that eating is about to happen, and the process of digestion begins. On the other hand, if we are looking at a television set, a computer screen, or even our not-so-smart smart phone while eating, our bodies may be getting mixed messages.

For example, if I am watching a horror movie or a crime drama, or having an argument while on the phone with someone, my stress hormones rise. This is normal. Unfortunately, when stress levels are high, digestion shuts down. To properly digest our food, we need to be present with the act of eating in a calm and relaxed manner.

The ears are another amazing set of sense organs. They allow us to hear and can heighten our awareness of the environment around us as well as the environment inside of us. If we are listening to something that is upsetting, or a noise that is unnerving, the body won't be relaxed and ready for digestion.

Do you remember when you were in high school and someone screeched fingernails or a metal object on the chalkboard? The sound could turn your stomach. Could you imagine eating while that sound is happening? Absolutely not! Make sure the environment where you are eating is harmonious to your ears. For example, you could be listening to the crackling sound of bacon being prepared, or onions and peppers sizzling in a frying pan. I'm just sayin'...

Let's move on to that beautiful thing that sits on the front of your face; your nose! It's a very powerful tool. No matter what size it is or what you may think of it (too big, too small, too crooked), your nose allows you to breathe in the aromas around you.

We can usually decipher from smell alone whether something is good for us. It's not 100 percent foolproof, but the majority of the time, your nose can tell you exactly what you need to know about whether to put a substance inside your body.

A client asked, "How would I know if something in my refrigerator is still good or if it has gone bad?"

I advised her to use her senses. "First, look at the food and see what it looks like. Does it have an odd color or uneven patches of color? Maybe some brown, green, orange, black, or white spots? Does it have a weird shiny glaze on top, or is there some fuzz growing on it?" And, then I told her, "Put your nose into the container and take a whiff. If your face recoils from that container in any way, it's a sure sign you shouldn't put that food into your mouth and eat it." You would be surprised how many people do not actually look at their food or smell it before it goes into their mouths. It's more common than you may think.

Most of us are rushing through meals and not connecting with our food or the fact that the food is actually going to become our bodies on a cellular level. We do not take time to connect with our senses, and we certainly do not take time to taste or chew our food, which can be a BIG problem for the digestive system.

I'll give you a personal example. Three times in the past two years, my husband suffered from food poisoning or had a negative reaction to something he ate after dining out at a restaurant or other eatery.

Each time he asked me to *taste* his food or he would put a little piece of it on my plate to share what he was eating. I would look at it. Then I would smell it. And then, I would put a small amount of it into my mouth to taste it. On each of the occasions he suffered from food poisoning, I said to him, "I don't like it. It's got an odd flavor," and I didn't eat any more of it.

My hubby, unfortunately, has a voracious appetite. Even if something tastes a little bit off, he'll bypass his senses to get that food into his stomach—not a good practice. But, he's not alone. Lots of people do this.

Just the other day, as he was gently nursing another stomachache, he finally said, "The next time we're out to eat, if you think the food tastes funny, do NOT let me eat it no matter how hungry I am!"

I said, "Okay. Until you can slow down and come to your senses, I'll be your guide on this."

There is a deep connection between your thyroid and the food you eat. The thyroid is the master communicator. It lets your body know exactly what's coming down the pipe. Just as I am communicating these words to you right now, the thyroid communicates internally to your body. It tells your body to speed up metabolism, slow down metabolism, store fat, release glucose, or lose weight, as well as many other functions. It's very good at its job.

We have to learn how to connect with our senses when healing the thyroid. First, take a moment to look at your food. Does it look appetizing? To determine if it is healthful, or not so healthful, just LOOK at it! It'll take only one or two seconds to scan your plate.

Then, smell that food. You don't have to put your whole face into the plate, but somehow get a whiff of it before it goes into your mouth. Put some on your fork and smell it. Aromas activate your salivary glands and digestive juices, and get your body ready for eating. Your sense of smell is also connected to your limbic system. The limbic system controls memory and emotions, and it's connected to the pituitary gland and hypothalamus, which control the release of hormones that affect our appetite, nervous system, body temperature, stress levels, and concentration.[47] Utilizing your sense of smell is essential for regulating your food intake and for letting you know whether or not something is going to nourish you.

I'm sure at one time or another in your life, you entered someone's home and the scent of home-cooked food made your mouth water or made you feel comfortable and safe. This is one of the reasons real estate agents sometimes bake a batch of cookies or bread if they are trying to sell a home. The aroma of baked goodies wafting in the air creates a sense of warmth, comfort, and well-being. Why do you think people line up outside bakeries when a new baked good is launched into the marketplace? We are all seeking comfort.

Our sense of smell can let us know whether something can physically and/or nutritionally support us on a deep level. When I was in my early thirties, I had "gone vegan" after reading some inspiring books about veganism. After two years of abstaining from all animal proteins and saturated fats, I began suffering from adrenal fatigue and muscle weakness.

When I finally contemplated eating meat again, I remember looking at the meat for a long time, and then smelling it. My mouth filled with saliva. It was the most interesting sensation. My glands became *very* active, and I was practically drooling!

That was a sign from my physical body that meat was the food I was supposed to eat at that time. My body was in a state of deficiency. Regardless of any information I had read in the vegan books or other "health-related" materials about meat being bad for health, my body was clearly saying something completely different. I honored my senses, gave my body what it needed, and my condition improved.

My friend, Jeannie, was a healthy vegan for thirteen years. When she got pregnant, she started having wild food cravings.

I advised her, "Relax and go with your cravings. The human body is very smart. When you're pregnant, all of your senses are naturally heightened. It's a form of protection and wisdom for the mother and growing fetus. Listen to your body, and give it what it needs."

One day Jeannie called me from a pay phone on a New York City street crying hysterically! In between sobs she said, "I am standing

47   http://www.dartmouth.edu/~rswenson/NeuroSci/chapter_9.html

in front of Burger King, and I am about to go inside and get a Whopper with cheese! You told me to listen to my body, and this is what my body said it needed!"

I said, "Great! I'm happy you're listening to your body, but please do NOT go into the fast food joint for your burger."

She said, "But I need it! It's what my body said."

I said, "I understand. But, please go to the nearest natural foods market or farmers market and pick up a pound of grass-fed ground beef and a big hunk of cheddar cheese. Then go home and make yourself a cheeseburger. You can sauté some onions and mushrooms, too. Plus put some pickles or sauerkraut on top to enhance digestion. That way you can have the food your body is craving, from naturally and humanely raised animals, and not feel guilty about it afterwards. Get the best quality meat, and let it nourish you and your baby on a deep level."

She did. And she felt healthier and stronger. She now has two beautiful children. She is no longer vegan, but is a conscious eater. Especially, about the meat she serves to her family.

Her scenario is not uncommon. Women, especially when pregnant, need to eat the most nutrient-dense and fatty foods to help nourish the endocrine system and the body as a whole. But many of us tend toward "more healthful" foods like salads and low-fat versions of things because we've been indoctrinated into a "dieting" mentality. That mindset can set up the body for thyroid disease and adrenal fatigue.

Our misguided thoughts about foods can sometimes override our good sense. I'm going to ask you to start tapping into your senses and bodily needs. Our senses are highly attuned to support the physical body; we just need to learn how to use them for healing.

That takes us to the next sense: our sense of taste. If we simply bite and swallow food, we won't be able to taste it, or digest it properly. If you don't "taste" food, you will always go back for second and third helpings. You won't feel satisfied after eating because you have bypassed the senses, and this can lead to overeating and being overweight.

Put food into your mouth and let it linger on your tongue for a moment. Then take the time to do something that most people do NOT do. You have to CHEW! That's why we have teeth. They are not just for smiling in pictures.

Most folks have forgotten, or were never taught, that they have to masticate their food with saliva to properly digest it. Lack of chewing is a recipe for digestive disaster!

When we chew food, we mix it with enzymes in our saliva that start the process of digestion where it's supposed to begin—in the mouth. If we don't chew our food, we risk indigestion, acid reflux, gastroesophageal reflux disease (GERD), irritable bowel syndrome (IBS), bloating, gas, weight gain, diabetes, and thyroid disease.

I had a client who was suffering from thyroid disease and had gained forty pounds in less than one year. That's a lot of weight! I asked her to focus on chewing her food.

She said, "Chewing? What kind of advice is that? I'm fifty-four years old! I'm not a little baby. I know how to chew my food."

I said, "Okay, I totally get that. But, just for fun, over the next couple of weeks I'd like you to focus on chewing your food. Let me know how many times you chew something before swallowing it. Experiment, and see if you can get to twenty-five chews per mouthful."

The next time we spoke, she said she couldn't believe it. She noticed she chewed only three or four times before swallowing. That means whole pieces of unchewed food were going down her throat and into her digestive system.

Our bodies cannot process whole pieces of food that way. Human beings are *not* designed like lions and tigers and bears. We cannot just bite and swallow our food, but that is what many people are doing. To heal any digestive troubles, including any autoimmune thyroid conditions, we absolutely NEED to chew our food.

When we chew, the parotid gland releases enzymes into the mouth. Those enzymes combine with saliva and help us break down our food so we can taste it and digest it.

Inez, a young client of mine who was in her early thirties, came to see me because she was diagnosed with hyperthyroidism. She had been on thyroid medication for five years, and her condition kept getting worse. The doctors wanted to remove her thyroid.

I asked Inez about her digestive health; she told me she had been suffering from acid reflux for over ten years. The reflux preceded her hyperthyroid condition, of course. I told her we needed to work on her digestive system to heal her condition. She told me she would run around the house finishing her chores while eating her meals, and her husband would yell at her to "sit down"!

I said, "Your hubby is absolutely correct. When you get home, give him a big hug. Please sit down while you are eating, slow down, and focus on chewing your food."

An interesting thing happened when she applied the simple knowledge of "how to eat." She told me that when she sat down, relaxed, and actually chewed her food, the reflux disappeared. It's not magic. It's simply the way we are designed.

When people chew their food, they naturally eat less, feel more satisfied, digest better, and lose weight. Chewing is like the miracle cure no one is talking about! It doesn't cost any money to chew food. You don't have to purchase any expensive supplements or digestive enzymes. It's FREE! You simply have to be conscious of chewing and activating the enzymes you were born with that help digest food.

The next time you sit down to eat, no matter what age you are, be conscious of whether you are chewing your food and activating your salivary glands. Check in and ask, "Do I swallow whole pieces of food when I'm eating?"

If you are eating soft foods like oatmeal or noodles, they can slide right down your throat, but they still need to be mixed with saliva to be digested properly. Drinking water or any other beverage with your meals can cause you to swallow whole pieces of food as well. It's very easy to take a bite of something and then a sip of wine, water, or other beverage, and then gulp... the whole piece of food goes right down the hatch!

The only liquid you want in your mouth when you are eating is your own saliva that contains the enzymes to start the process of digestion where it is supposed to begin: in the mouth, not in the stomach. This doesn't mean you cannot have a drink with your meals. It just means to be conscious that you are NOT using your beverages to gulp down whole pieces of unchewed food. The only people who can gulp their food are babies, and that's because they don't have any teeth. Plus, the adults feeding them make sure that baby food is pureed before it goes into the baby's mouth.

Which brings me to another digestive disaster: formula fed babies! Mother's milk is imperative to the health of the baby. Mother's milk contains the colostrum and antibodies needed to colonize the baby's intestines to help that little human begin building its immune system. Without that first coating of mother's milk in the intestines, the baby may suffer from many illnesses throughout its lifetime, including thyroid disease.

I was born in the late 1960s, and at that time, nutritional science convinced moms across America that their breast milk was inferior to the super vitamin-enhanced baby formula created in laboratories.

That was a HUGE mistake! Today, we know that formula-fed babies have higher rates of ALL diseases across the board including asthma, allergies, diabetes, cancer, thyroid disease, and digestive ailments like Crohn's, colitis, and IBS.[48]

First and foremost, many of those baby formulas contain soy. Most folks already know how detrimental unfermented soy is to the thyroid. For those of you who do *not* know, I'll cover that information in the food chapter.

Secondly, for those of you who were formula-fed babies, do NOT get angry at your mom! She thought she was doing the best thing for you. She followed the nutritional science and not the design of her beautiful body.

Once again, we need to understand that the human body is perfectly designed, and that includes the breasts. Not only are they beautiful, but they also serve as built-in baby bottles to feed the baby exactly what it needs to thrive.

Colostrum that is found in breast milk in the first feedings for the baby works as a natural, 100 percent safe vaccine; the immune agents and antibodies give the baby protection from external germs that enter into the throat, lungs, and intestines. Colostrum plays a key role in the baby's intestinal tract. It seals the permeable holes of the intestines and prevents foreign bodies from entering the intestines. Colostrum prevents jaundice and also acts as a laxative by loosening meconium, the baby's first stool.

---

48   University of Washington Medical Research Center

Colostrum contains high concentrations of leucocytes, the protective white cells that destroy disease-causing bacteria and viruses.[49] [50]

Thanks to colostrum, breast-fed babies begin their life on planet Earth in a much stronger and more healthful way. But, have no fear. If you've been formula fed like me, you can still support your intestines and nourish your thyroid. Remember to be patient and loving with your body while you are getting to know it better. Your digestive system and immunity may need extra loving care and attention from you a little more often.

Another reason the digestive system may not be functioning properly is prescription medications. Prescription drugs like oral contraceptives, acid blockers, diuretics, proton pump inhibitors, diabetes medications, and antibiotics are the top offenders contributing to nutrient deficiencies. Those drugs can deplete or block the absorption of folic acid, coenzyme Q10, calcium, iron, zinc, magnesium, and vitamins B6, B12, D, and C.[51]

If you're taking prescription medications, make sure you research the contraindications and side effects associated with them. Some of the symptoms of thyroid disease that you may be experiencing could stem from nutritional deficiencies and an inability to digest food from taking prescription medications.

Acid-suppressing medications for acid reflux and GERD inhibit our ability to absorb nutrients, especially vitamins D and B12 and zinc, which are essential for healthy thyroid and endocrine system function. As you've already discovered, there are easy ways to stop acid reflux and GERD, and it starts with chewing your gosh darn food!

The overuse of antibiotics destroys intestinal flora and can inhibit our ability to digest. I'm not saying antibiotics are bad. They're not. They can actually save your life if you need them. What I'm talking about is the overuse and abuse of antibiotics.

Antibiotics are given to factory-farmed animals in their daily food rations to help keep them alive (and fatten them up) while they are confined in highly stressful and unhealthful environments. The constant stream of antibiotics in their feed creates drug-resistant and fatal strains

---

49   http://www.askdrsears.com/topics/feeding-eating/breastfeeding/why-breast-is-best/how-human-milk-protects-babies-illness
50   http://www.nrdc.org/breastmilk/benefits.asp
51   http://www.alive.com/articles/view/23097/drug-induced_nutritional_deficiency

of bacteria that are being passed into humans.[52] On top of that scary scenario, we humans are being prescribed antibiotics for everything from acne to colds and toenail fungus. It's ridiculous!

Stop taking antibiotics for every little sniffle you encounter. You may be setting yourself up for a digestive system that is overgrown with bad bacteria, which can lead to autoimmune conditions.

People suffering from Graves' disease and Hashimoto's thyroiditis always tell me the same thing, "My doctor told me my condition is incurable because it's autoimmune."

Doctors are correct in their understanding. They learned in medical school that autoimmune conditions are incurable and are treated with medications that suppress bodily symptoms. Unfortunately, that treatment can exacerbate the situation and make the condition worse![53]

Thankfully, there are many natural health practitioners, health coaches, and integrative/functional medicine professionals who understand something completely different about healing the body. They understand that discovering the root cause of ANY autoimmune condition starts by diving into the digestive system. If the digestive system is overrun by rogue bacteria and viruses, the immune system becomes compromised.

According to the National Institutes of Health and the United States National Library of Medicine: "There are more than eighty identified autoimmune diseases. Multiple factors are thought to contribute to the development of immune response to self, including genetics, age, and environment. In particular, viruses, bacteria and other infectious pathogens are the major postulated environmental triggers of autoimmunity."[54]

I recommend following an herbal protocol that could include black walnut hull and wormwood to help get rid of bad bugs and parasites. We will cover some of these herbs in depth in the chapter "Helpful Herbs and Botanical Medicine."

Let's move on to mercury and how it can affect the digestive system. I don't know which rocket scientist thought putting one of the

52   http://opinionator.blogs.nytimes.com/2013/07/09/breeding-bacteria-on-factory-farms/?_php=true&_type=blogs&_r=0
53   http://drhyman.com/blog/2010/07/30/how-to-stop-attacking-yourself-9-steps-to-heal-autoimmune-disease/#close
54   http://www.ncbi.nlm.nih.gov/pmc/articles/PMC2665673/

most toxic substances on the planet into the teeth was a good idea, but he certainly wasn't using his head! Mercury in our teeth has done more damage to our health than we can ever imagine, or that the American Dental Association would ever admit.

Mercury damages the tissues around it. It starts with the tissues that are closest first, and then it moves to other parts of the body. The sublingual and parotid glands are the first parts to be affected by mercury in the mouth, and then the thyroid.[55] Other parts of the body affected by mercury include the eyes, sinuses, and the brain, as well as the digestive system, nervous system, and the kidneys.[56]

Mercury toxicity contributes to renal failure, infertility, tremors, digestive dysfunctions, autoimmune diseases including Graves' and Hashimoto's, hearing loss, memory loss, Alzheimer's disease, cognitive impairment, and hallucinations.

In the 1800s, the term "mad as a hatter" came from the hat-making industry. Mercury was used in the production of felt, which, at that time, was used to make hats. People working in the hat-making industry were exposed to mercury on a daily basis. Many of them developed early dementia and the saying "mad as a hatter" was born.

I had a client who had been suffering from thyroid disease for over twenty-five years. Margaret came to see me for a consultation and began rattling off her symptoms: she couldn't think straight, was always lost or in a fog, was paranoid, and suffering from insomnia and tremors. She said, "I feel like I am losing my mind."

When she opened her mouth to speak, I could see that almost ALL of her teeth were filled with mercury. I couldn't believe it! She must've had twenty or more fillings in her mouth. With all of that mercury, it may not matter how healthful her diet and lifestyle were, her thyroid and parotid glands could continue getting damaged with each bite of food. It may take quite a long time to heal her condition, possibly seven years or longer, depending on whether her kidneys and adrenals were damaged by that mouthful of mercury as well, which is a strong possibility.

If you have many mercury amalgams and you are suffering from thyroid disease, I would suggest getting them SAFELY removed. And, I

55   http://www.naturalblaze.com/2013/04/mercury-fillings-and-missing-link-in.html
56   http://www.mercola.com/article/mercury/mercury_elimination.htm

want to emphasize "safely"! If you get mercury removed by someone who is not qualified, you could be exposed to toxic levels of mercury when it is extracted. I've had many clients tell me they have had mercury removed, and they immediately began suffering from toxicity that lasted one year or longer.

Do some research to make sure your dentist is using the best methods possible to safely extract the mercury. And, keep in mind that even if it is done safely, you could still be exposed to traces of mercury. Do NOT get any mercury removed if you are pregnant or nursing. That could lead to birth defects and be disastrous to the health of your baby.

I had about ten mercury fillings in my mouth by the time I was twenty years old. I still have a few left. My thyroid is normal today, even with the remaining mercury fillings. It's possible that the excessive amount of mercury I was originally exposed to was one of the contributing factors to my hyperthyroid disease.

Eventually, I may have the remaining mercury removed, but I would only do it one tooth at a time. Many dentists recommend removing all the mercury at the same time—I don't think that's a wise idea. The body needs time to process and recover at a slow and gentle pace. In the meantime, you could use delicious foods, like garlic, cilantro, and sea vegetables, that bind with mercury and naturally excrete it from the body.

If you have root canals in your mouth and you have any type of cancer, including thyroid cancer, you may want to think about getting those teeth extracted. Root canals may have been a good idea with good intentions, but this has also proven to be a bad idea. Root canals are a breeding ground for bacteria and disease. They have been linked with heart disease, kidney disease, arthritis, autoimmune conditions, and breast and thyroid cancers.[57]

I had many root canals in my mouth. A couple of the root canals rotted away, and I had one tooth extracted. It's traumatizing to lose teeth! I still have a couple of root canals and may eventually get those teeth extracted as well, depending on my health. If I ever get diagnosed with cancer, those root canals are coming out.

---

57   http://articles.mercola.com/sites/articles/archive/2012/02/18/dangers-of-root-canaled-teeth.aspx

Let's take another look at mercury because it's not just in our mouths. We also get mercury from vaccines, which can be a BIG problem. More and more vaccinations are popping up every year.

When I was growing up, we got vaccinated for mumps, measles, rubella, polio, whooping cough, and tetanus. It was about five or six vaccinations. Nowadays kids can get as many as forty-five doses of various vaccination shots by the time they are teenagers.[58] That is a lot for their growing immune systems to handle!

A few years ago, the Center For Disease Control and other government organizations decided to remove mercury from most vaccines. That was a pretty smart decision. Unfortunately, now many of the vaccines around the world that kids are being injected with have aluminum instead of mercury. Lord have mercy! It seems we just do one dangerous thing after another.

Aluminum is one of those metals that accumulate in the soft tissues, especially in the brain. Aluminum is a known neurotoxin that can lead to long-term brain inflammation. There is overwhelming evidence that chronic immune inflammation in your brain contributes to multiple sclerosis, Alzheimer's disease, and Parkinson's disease.[59]

As it relates to thyroid health, metal toxicity in the body contributes to endocrine dysfunctions, hyperthyroidism, and renal failure. Please limit the numbers of vaccinations for both you and your children. No one really needs the chicken pox vaccine, do they?

I personally have NOT had a flu shot since 1998. Instead I get a natural flu vaccine every year by interacting with people who actually have the flu. They sneeze, "Ahhh choo," and I say, "God Bless you." After that, my body immediately begins building immunity to that person's flu, unless my immunity has been compromised in some way.

Something to keep in mind is that the flu mutates every year. It's never the same strain of flu as it was the year before. That means when you get a flu shot, you're actually getting last year's flu, not this year's flu. I would much rather get the current year's flu. It just makes more sense.

---

58   http://www.cdc.gov/vaccines/schedules/hcp/imz/child-adolescent.html
59   http://articles.mercola.com/sites/articles/archive/2009/01/27/mercury-in-vaccines-was-replaced-with-something-even-more-toxic.aspx

It's time to move on to some other chemicals that can disrupt the functioning of our internal environment. Perflourinated chemicals (PFOA) are used to make nonstick cookware. Higher concentrations of PFOAs in the human body have been directly linked with thyroid disease, infertility, and bladder, kidney, and testicular cancers.[60] I understand that nonstick pans may be easier to work with and much easier to clean, but they also pose a danger to your reproductive system and your thyroid. Use good old-fashioned stainless steel pots and pans, cast iron or ceramic cookware, and earthenware pots—these are more traditional cooking vessels.

Plus, as you'll learn in the food section of this book, fat acts as a natural lubricant for your body. With the addition of saturated fat into your diet, you can use some of it in your pans to prevent food from sticking.

If you DO have nonstick pans, you can still use them, just don't EVER use metal on them! Use wood or plastic utensils. If you use metal, you could accidentally scrape the nonstick coating on those pans, and it will find its way into your digestive system.

If you have any nonstick pans that are already scraped and damaged, toss them out. Any healthful recipe that you cook in a damaged nonstick pan becomes an unhealthful dish, no matter how good your ingredients are.

Now, some of you may be thinking, "What am I supposed to do? I cook with nonstick pans. I sit in front of a computer all day. I talk on the cell phone. I cook my food in the microwave. There are endocrine-disrupting chemicals in the food and in the water. There's mercury in my mouth, and maybe some root canals in there too. I'm doomed!"

Wrong! I'm here to remind you that no matter what is going on right now, you are still alive. WHEW! Pat yourself on the back and give yourself a hug. Whatever you have been doing up until now has gotten you here, to this point in your life, reading this book.

Human beings are resilient creatures. We are highly adaptable. As long as you are alive and breathing, you can improve any condition on some level, whether it's physical, energetic (vibrational), emotional, or spiritual. Your strength is going to come from the fact that you are *still here* and you are in the process of learning something new. You are in the process of healing.

60 http://www.cancer.org/cancer/cancercauses/othercarcinogens/athome/teflon-and-perflurooctanoic-acid--pfoa

I know you may be suffering from symptoms that totally stink, and you may be feeling uncomfortable, but as often as possible, when you wake up in the morning, say to yourself, "Wow! I'm still here! Today is going to be a good day."

With every chapter you read, you are gaining a new understanding of how your body may have gotten out of balance, and you're also learning how to set things right again. Now it's time to take a look at some of the ways we can rebalance the body, support the endocrine system, and heal your thyroid condition.

CHAPTER 7
Recharging Our Batteries

It's time to discover some of the many ways we can recharge our batteries to increase our energy, heal underlying conditions, and best support our thyroid. In a previous chapter, I asked you to look at your computer and cell phone. They are running on electrical energy. They need to use batteries, be plugged in to an energy source, or be recharged from an energy source. These technologies will simply not run without connecting to some type of power.

Human beings also have to connect to a power source to keep running efficiently and healthfully. But, most of us are not connecting because we don't know what that source is or what it means to connect.

The first and most important energy source for us to connect to is Earth. The BIG round ball, suspended in the universe, that we are living on is amazing. Besides providing an abundance of food for its inhabitants, Earth is also a powerful source of renewable energy. Before I give you the crunchy granola version of why we need to connect to Earth, I'm going to share some scientific data.

In the 1950s, a German physics professor named Winfried Otto Schumann discovered frequencies that resonate within and around Earth. Many scientists, including the bigwigs at NASA, have tested these energetic frequencies and confirmed that they do exist and do have an effect on human health.[61] Those electromagnetic frequencies found emanating in Earth are called Schumann resonances, after the physicist who discovered it. There are many more electromagnetic fields and geomagnetic fields resonating in Earth as well.

Professor Rütger Wever, from the Max Planck Institute for Behavioral Physiology, and his associate Jürgen Aschoff built an underground bunker that completely screened out Earth's various frequencies. For the experiments, student volunteers lived in the bunker for weeks at a time. They were sealed into an environment that was devoid of ALL of Earth's natural frequencies. The Professor and his associate noted that throughout their time in the bunker, the students' circadian rhythms diverged and they suffered emotional distress and severe migraine headaches. The Professor then reintroduced Earth's frequencies into the sealed environment, and the results were

61   http://www.glcoherence.org/monitoring-system/earth-rhythms.html

astonishing. After only a brief exposure to the frequencies of Earth, the volunteers' health stabilized.[62]

This demonstrated a direct link between humans and Earth. It's interesting that we are so disconnected from Earth that we need scientific testing to prove we're actually connected, energetically, to the planet we're living on.

We are so *removed* from Earth, in fact, that we can easily destroy it and pollute it without thinking about how it will affect us. We live here on the planet; of course we are connected to it in a deep way. It's basic common sense. Earth is our home and our source for organic life.

That particular experiment with Professor Wever and the students in the sealed bunker lasted only a few weeks. Many of us have gone far longer than that being disconnected from the frequencies of Earth. We live and work in sealed environments that can cut us off from, or disrupt the flow of, the natural frequencies we need to be exposed to on a daily basis. And, as you've learned, we are also surrounded by multiple technologies that can disrupt the flow of energy in the human body. It's no wonder we're exhausted, sick, and suffering from emotional distress. We're unwittingly disrupting our energy flow and cutting ourselves off from one of our main sources of energy.

But, you're in luck. I'm going to show you how to reestablish your connection to the amazing pulses in Earth and increase your energy to generate healthy cells and potentially heal your condition.

There are many consumer products on the market today that promise to help get you grounded and reconnected to Earth: earthing mats, amethyst crystal beds, and other fun stuff like that. I think those products are great and can possibly help you feel better. But, there is absolutely, positively NO substitution for actually getting outside into nature and connecting directly to Earth itself. As an added bonus, while you are outside, you will be exposed to trees, air, sunshine, and everything your body needs to thrive. And the best part? It's all FREE! As an inhabitant of planet Earth, the universe has provided it for you. All you have to do is step outside your house or your office, and go get it.

---

62   http://www.collective-evolution.com/2013/12/19/experiment-proves-why-staying-in-tune-with-the-earths-pulse-is-key-to-our-well-being/

I always suggest that clients and students take a *daily* walk in nature, or go to a city park where they are surrounded by trees. Trees are directly rooted into Earth and vibrate healing frequencies.

There is a wonderful relationship between trees and all living creatures. We breathe out carbon, and trees take in carbon and give us oxygen, which we breathe in. It's a perfect symbiotic relationship. We support each other and contribute to each other's well-being and survival on this planet.

If you're ever feeling low on energy, chronically fatigued, and generally unwell, it would be wise to get outside and surround yourself with trees and nature. It can naturally improve your air quality and oxygen levels.

People suffering from any type of depression or melancholy should literally go out and hug a tree. I'm not even kidding. I'm a bona fide tree hugger. I love trees. We even have many scientific studies proving the *loss* of trees has a negative impact on physiological health. "The loss of trees to the emerald ash borer increased mortality related to cardiovascular and lower-respiratory-tract illness."[63]

If you're not going to hug a tree, at least just sit underneath one to absorb some of its healing energy. Bring a picnic lunch to any park, and enjoy eating it while sitting underneath the canopy of a majestic tree. You'll feel highly energized and alert. Or you'll fall fast asleep, especially if your body is telling you that it really needs to rest.

Keep in mind that the frequency of Earth is still present underneath cities, but it is competing with many of the man-made frequencies we've created, like subways, phone wires, and internet connections. Unfortunately, many of our man-made frequencies are the ones that have been slowly breaking us down, destroying the integrity of our cells, and draining our energy reserves.

A group of teenage girls in Denmark conducted a science experiment that won them top honors. The girls noticed that if they slept with their cell phones near their heads at night, they had difficulty concentrating at school the next day. They were curious and wanted to know if there was a connection. The girls designed a science experiment that would test the effects of man-made radiation on plants. They placed

---

63   http://donovan.hnri.info/Studies/donovan_et_al.EAB.pdf

six trays filled with garden cress seeds into a room without radiation and six trays of the garden cress seeds into another room next to two Wi-Fi routers that emitted the same type of radiation as a cellphone. Over the next two weeks, the girls observed, measured, weighed, and photographed their results. By the end of their experiment, the results were obvious. The cress seeds placed near the Wi-Fi routers had not matured, and many of them were dead. The cress seeds planted in the second room, away from the routers, sprouted and thrived. The experiment earned the teenagers top honors in a regional science competition.[64]

If you are seeking to grow and change the quality of your cells, as when you're healing from thyroid cancer or any type of cancer, it's important to gain some distance from the man-made frequencies as much as possible and get into nature as often as possible. We all have Wi-Fi routers in our homes and workplaces, and they are constantly emitting low levels of radiation. Think about your body as being filled with seeds (cells) that you want to grow to be healthy and strong. There are easy ways to make that happen. For example, take this wise book you're reading right now and go sit under a tree for a couple of hours. It can make a big difference in the growth and health of your cells.

Another way to increase energy is to help the body discharge toxins and waste through normal bodily functions. If you're not discharging waste properly your body can, and will, become toxic. When it comes to healing thyroid conditions, including thyroid cancer, you want to rid bodily waste on a daily basis.

We naturally discharge waste through various detoxification pathways in the body: through breathing, we release carbon dioxide via the respiratory system; through defecating, we excrete solid waste and toxins via the excretory system, and through urinating, we release liquid waste from the urinary system. Through the integumentary system, which includes skin, we release waste through sweating.

Breathing and getting rid of waste through our lungs comes pretty easily for most folks, except those who have asthma or other respiratory disorders. Unfortunately, many of us—not just the asthmatics— breathe up into our chest. This is not a healthful way to breathe because it limits the amount of oxygen we can bring to our cells and can simultaneously create fear and stress. Take a breathing class, yoga class, or

64   http://www.naturalnews.com/043238_wi-fi_routers_radiation_plant_growth.html

meditation class to learn proper breathing techniques. In the "A Deeper Truth About Thyroid Health" chapter, I'll share with you some easy breathing exercises.

To urinate and release our bowels on a daily basis, we need good quality food that has been chewed well, and we need to drink water. As we move our physical bodies with exercise, we naturally release sweat and oil. This is all basic common sense. Once again, I want to remind you that the body is perfectly designed. If we give it what it needs, it does its job of naturally eliminating our waste.

Now here's the interesting part. If I told you to hold your breath and stop breathing, would you? Of course not! If you did that you would pass out. Stopping your breath would be detrimental to your life. And, if I told you to stop peeing and pooping on a regular basis, would you? Of course not! You want that waste out of your body—it becomes toxic if we don't eliminate it in a timely manner. But, if I told you to stop sweating because sweating is gross, would you? Think about that for a moment. Many of us are doing that on a daily basis. We use antiperspirants to stop the body from doing what it is designed to do... SWEAT! This is terribly unhealthful for us. Many of those antiperspirants also contain aluminum that is absorbed into your body every time you put it onto your skin. Metal toxicity contributes to thyroid disease, as well as to Alzheimer's.

Please keep in mind that you would never use an antipooperator to stop your body from pooping. So I am going to suggest that you do NOT use an antiperspirant to stop your body from sweating. You need to sweat.

Don't get me wrong. I'm not suggesting that you do not use any deodorant. Please do! I don't want you to lose friends and lovers over a little bit of natural odor. There are many deodorants that can help you mask the odor of sweat without stopping the process of sweating. What I want you to do is begin trusting and honoring the way your body is designed. Unless you have been born without sweat glands, please sweat.

I had a client who didn't sweat for almost twenty years! She had a lump in her breast, and the first thing I suggested was that she STOP wearing antiperspirant. She needed to have the area near her breast flowing and releasing on a daily basis. She stopped using the antiperspirant, and it took her body eight months to begin sweating again! That's how clogged her system was. Contrary to what the advertisements for antiperspirants tell you, sweating is good. It helps your body release waste.

You can also purposely induce sweating by exercising or sitting in a sauna or steam room to help aid your body's detoxification process. Promoting sweating has been used as a detoxification and healing practice by many cultures around the world.

Here's an analogy for you about toxicity. If I chose NOT to take out the garbage in my house, it would pile up all over the place. My home would be a breeding ground for bacteria and pathogens to thrive and grow. Your physical body is the home you are living in. Take the garbage out!

I would also suggest that no matter how healthy you think you are, you are still living in a toxic environment and need to do some type of intentional cleansing and/or fasting. Every year I do a liver cleanse and encourage my clients and students to do the same.

If the liver is congested or overburdened with eliminating toxins, the thyroid will be out of balance. The liver detoxifies and moves the blood. Impaired liver function leads to increased estrogen levels and decreased T4 to T3 conversion. The liver is a detoxification organ, and if it's not working optimally, your body simply won't function properly.

In Traditional Chinese Medicine, the liver and gallbladder meridians correlate with the season of spring. In the springtime, it would be wise to reduce animal fats and proteins as well as do some type of fasting to support the healing and renewal of the liver and gallbladder.

It seems religions around the world and traditional healing therapies have this commonality as well. Some examples include the Orthodox Greeks who fast from animal foods for up to seven weeks during the spring. They abstain from foods that contain animals with red blood (meats, poultry, game), products that come from animals with red blood (milk, cheese, eggs), and fish and seafood. Wine and olive oil are also restricted. Fasting is serious business! Imagine life with no olive oil?

The Catholics fast for forty days prior to Easter. This fast includes eating overall lighter meals and abstaining from meat on Fridays.

Many cultures around the world use some type of cleansing or fasting process, specifically in the spring, to help lift the heaviness of winter—physically, emotionally, and spiritually. If we don't purposely cleanse or fast as spring arrives, the body naturally begins cleansing itself of excess oils, fats, salt, and animal proteins by releasing a flu or cold. Some people may also suffer from odd aches and pains during the spring months (and often throughout the year) and they don't know why. This can be a sign of liver congestion.

We can aid the body through a natural cleansing and detoxification process by eating light meals of steamed, sautéed, blanched, and raw foods, by eating less food overall, by eliminating animal products for a specific period of time, or by abstaining from food entirely. The springtime, I believe, is the best time of year to go vegan or vegetarian for a few weeks. It can highly benefit the health of your liver.

Another way to increase energy and recharge your battery is to incorporate ancient healing exercises. When I was suffering from thyroid disease and couldn't lose weight, I was going to the gym three to four times per week, endlessly climbing that StairMaster to nowhere for forty-five minutes to an hour. It seemed the harder I exercised, the more stubborn my weight was. It was ridiculous!

What I didn't know then was that I needed to balance my exercise routine with relaxing and recharging exercises as well, otherwise I would burn myself out. These recharging exercises include ancient exercises that have been around for thousands of years: Tai Chi, QiGong, and yoga.

Yoga includes breath control, simple meditative movements, stretching, and specific body postures that have been traditionally used for health and relaxation and to activate and energize the body chakras. I'll go deeper into what the chakras are and how they relate to thyroid health in another chapter.

Also, when I'm talking about yoga, I need to clarify that I'm talking about simple gentle hatha yoga. I'm not referring to strenuous exercise yoga, which is what folks experience in many of the gyms, and I'm certainly not talking about vigorous HOT yoga that is practiced in an excessively hot and humid room.

I had a client who was suffering from hypothyroidism and extreme fatigue; she said she was "always thirsty." Maryanne just couldn't seem to satisfy her thirst no matter how much water she drank. That could indicate the beginning stage of diabetes, but her thirst was due to something else.

When I asked her what type of exercise she did, she told me she was going to hot yoga four to five times per week because she wanted to "sweat the excess weight out of her system." Hot yoga may work for some folks, especially if their bodies are in a state of excess, or they need to sweat out toxins. But, if they are suffering from adrenal fatigue that leads to hypothyroidism like Maryanne was, hot yoga may not be the best choice.

Exercising in a room that is 105°F (or more) five times per week can be both stressful and extremely draining to the physical body, as well as make you very thirsty. When Maryanne made the simple switch from strenuous hot yoga to gentle hatha yoga, it made all the difference in the world to both her weight and her insatiable thirst.

Keep in mind, I am not telling you NOT to do hot yoga. I want you to begin understanding your own physical condition and then make the appropriate adjustments to heal your body. That's what you are doing here: learning about your condition and ways to possibly heal it, one chapter at a time.

Every body is unique. What works for one person may not work for another. Experimentation and reflection are needed for healing any condition.

Tai Chi, a form of martial arts, and QiGong, a traditional healing system of exercise, are also fantastic ways to rejuvenate and energize the body. With QiGong, you are using your breath and specific movements to harness energy from the universe and Earth and draw it into your system to circulate it throughout your body. The movements are gentle and slow like a form of meditation.

With many of these ancient exercises and healing practices, you would also use visualization to pull energy up from Earth and down from the universe to use in your body. In order for us to thrive, we humans need both Earth energy radiating from below us and universal energy radiating from above us. We are literally between Heaven and Earth.

Scientists have discovered there is energy in Earth that we cannot function healthfully without. Before long, they will do their scientific experiments once again to discover what the ancient people already knew: there is energy available to us emanating from the entire universe (the spaces above us, below us and all around us) that we also simply cannot live healthfully without.

Some open-minded scientists are already light years ahead of their contemporaries. "Human physiological rhythms and behaviors are synchronized with solar and geomagnetic activity, so fluctuations in the earth and sun's magnetic fields can affect virtually every circuit in human as well as any biological systems."[65]

The science is getting closer to understanding the invisible energies emanating from Earth, the sun, and the entire universe, and how they affect us. But, I would suggest you NOT wait for mainstream science to catch up with what our indigenous ancestors already knew. Start doing some type of ancient healing exercises on a *daily* basis to increase your energy. Google it, watch it on YouTube, get a DVD, or take a class – just do it! Rejuvenating exercises are needed in the world because we are constantly on the go and always expending our energy. Go, go, go, go, go! It's not healthful. It's exhausting. And, your thyroid and adrenals are feeling that drain.

This doesn't mean that I do not want you to go for a run or do cardiovascular exercise. I totally do! Running, jogging, rebounding, and other cardiovascular exercises help your body sweat and breathe and improve your lymphatic function and circulation, all of which promotes the discharge of waste. We totally need that!

We need to learn how to balance our exercise routines so we have some relaxing and rejuvenating exercises that enhance energy as well as high-energy exercises that expend energy. Switch up your routine to include yoga, stretching, a daily walk, QiGong, running, weight training, and anything else that makes you happy.

Every morning I do some type of stretching (meridian stretching) or yoga for fifteen to twenty minutes, plus I incorporate energy exercises like QiGong. It takes only a small percentage of time in the morning to charge my batteries for the entire day. I do it because it feels good, and I know as soon as I get out into the world, I will be expending energy. By doing a morning practice, I ensure I'm fully charged before starting my day.

Here's a good quote by Albert Einstein, super genius, to help you understand energy, "Energy cannot be created or destroyed, it can only be changed from one form to another."

Energy is everywhere. It's in Earth, it's in the food, it's in the universe. We are energy, and we are surrounded by energy. By learning

---

65   https://www.heartmath.org/research/global-coherence/

some ancient exercises, you have the golden opportunity to harness that energy and change it into a usable form in your body. I highly encourage you to learn how to access the energy in the world around you and draw it into your body for healing purposes.

Another way to increase energy and rejuvenate your body for healing is massage. Some people think getting a massage is extravagant or indulgent, but the truth is bodywork has been around for thousands of years, and there's a reason for that. It is highly therapeutic!

Massage improves circulation, reduces stress hormones, eases pain, and boosts immunity by moving lymphatic fluids. Get your physical body into the hands of a professional, and let him or her move your energy around for you.

I go for some type of massage or bodywork at least two times per month, depending on my workload. Receiving a massage gives me the opportunity to relax and let go of my need to do everything. I put myself into someone else's hands, literally! There are energetic points on my back that need to be stimulated. I could certainly attempt acting like a bear and rub my back up against a tree, but I'd much rather lie down, chill out, breathe deeply, and have a knowledgeable practitioner massage those points for me.

You don't have to go to a fancy spa and spend hundreds of dollars for a massage, unless of course you have the money and you want to. Research massage practitioners in your area, and find someone whose energy you like, because this person's energy will be moving your energy. There is always some transference of energy between people who are working together, so make sure you get a good vibe from the person who is going to be working on you.

When I was researching massage therapists and bodyworkers in my area, I tried out ten different people before I found someone I really liked. I've been seeing her regularly now for almost ten years. We are in an energetic relationship, so to speak. Go find someone you like and get some bodywork. That means go out and get massaged by a bunch of different people. The research alone is going to make you happy.

Another one of my favorite ways to enhance energy is with a good night's sleep. Sleep rejuvenates us, rebuilds our bodies, and lets us restore our life force. We need adequate sleep to heal. Whether it's adrenal fatigue, thyroid disease, or any other condition in the physical or the emotional body, we absolutely need sleep. Unfortunately, most of us are not getting enough of it. Or, we're not getting good quality sleep when we do get it.

The first thing I'm going to suggest is that you remove from your sleeping area any technology that emits nonionizing radiation or low-level electromagnetic frequencies. These technologies interrupt our sleep patterns.

That means, take the television OUT of the bedroom! This will not only improve your sleep, but it can probably improve your relationship with your significant other as well. You won't have a television to distract you. You'll look over at the other person in the bed and say, "Hmm, well... there's nothing to really do in here... maybe we could try a little hanky-panky." Or, maybe you'll look over at that person and actually have a conversation, "Hello person that I share my life with. It's nice to see you here." Taking the television out of your bedroom can help you connect more deeply with your partner on many levels.

If you're a single person and no one is in the bed with you, without a television you can finally read the book that's been sitting on your night table for the past two years because you haven't had time for it. Or you can start journaling at night to get to know yourself better.

Many substantial things can happen when we take the technology, including computers and cellphones, out of the bedroom. As you've already learned, these technologies emit light directly into your pineal gland. That can knock your natural circadian rhythm out of sync and interrupt the body's ability to release melatonin that helps you sleep. It would be wise to stop using the computer and cell phone at least three hours before bed. Give your endocrine system, your nervous system, and brain some time to relax and decompress.

Another way to ensure a good night's rest is not to eat directly before bed. A three-hour window of no food in your stomach before lying down to sleep would be ideal. Going to bed while your body is still digesting food inhibits the body's regenerative abilities. The body starts the process of healing and restoration at night while you're sleeping. The major restorative functions in the body, like muscle growth, tissue repair, protein synthesis, and growth hormone, release during sleep.[66] If you have food in your belly, your body is working on digestion, not restoration. Do you eat before going to bed? If yes, please stop it!

---

66   http://healthysleep.med.harvard.edu/healthy/matters/benefits-of-sleep/why-do-we-sleep

Getting to bed at a decent hour is imperative to healing. Human beings need to sleep with the moon and wake with the sun. When we sleep with the cycle of the moon, it helps support and heal the kidneys, as well as the rest of the body. This is ancient healing wisdom.

Modern science confirms that people working the nightshift have higher rates of heart disease, stroke, diabetes, gastrointestinal disorders, infertility, and cancer.[67] It's called the graveyard shift for a reason!

I've had many clients tell me they just can't get to bed by 11:00 p.m. They insist they are "night owls." Yeah, that might actually work for an owl because it is physically designed to function better in the dark of night. Owls have an acute sense of hearing, as well as very large forward facing eyes with stereoscopic binocular vision that allows them to see one-hundred times better than humans—especially at night.[68] So unless you have supersonic hearing and HUGE eyes that can see in the dark, shut off the man-made technologies and get to bed by 11:00 p.m. or earlier. "Whoooo me?" Yes you!

Many clients who were suffering from chronic digestive problems and allergies magically cleared up most of their symptoms once they began going to bed at a decent hour. It's not really magic. It's just the way the human body is designed to function best: active during the day, sleeping during the night.

Other energy sources for us to tap into are our environment and our food. In upcoming chapters, we are going to go in depth about the various types of food and how they affect our health. Right now, we're going to look at how our *environment* can affect our food choices.

In each environment and climate of the world, there are various types of ecosystems. Each of those ecosystems is inhabited by specific plant and animal species that thrive in those environments. I'm going to use trees as an example.

In a desert environment, cacti grow and thrive. In tropical and subtropical environments, palm trees, coconuts trees, and banana trees thrive. Although those are both hot environments, their climates are very different. One is hot and dry, and the other is hot and wet. These two environments have distinctive ecosystems.

---

67   http://www.webmd.com/sleep-disorders/excessive-sleepiness-10/shift-work?page=2
68   http://www.owlpages.com/articles.php?section=Owl+Physiology&title=Vision

In a temperate climate, maple, oak, birch, and sycamore trees thrive, and in the winter, lose their leaves and seemingly become barren. In a frigid or cold climate, spruce, fir, and pine trees thrive and keep their needles all winter long. As you can see, these two environments are different, and the things that grow in them vary as well.

If I were to take a cactus from Mexico and plant it on top of the snowy mountains in Canada, it would never be able to survive in that environment. Even though a cactus might look really good up there among the pines, it doesn't have the right elements to sustain its survival.

Each ecosystem has exactly the right amount of sunshine, rainfall, and specific types of soil for its plant species to thrive. And every animal within that entire ecosystem is also in harmony with the plants and is thriving as well. Except, it seems, for us modern humans. We have given ourselves all of the creature comforts of a warm home and shelter, but we have neglected to keep ourselves in alignment with our surrounding environment.

We have disconnected from the natural environment and the ecosystem we live in by eating plants and foods that are grown all over the world in many different types of climates and regions. This may seem like a good idea, but it's actually not good for our physical bodies or for our environment.

Where I live in the northeastern United States, palm trees, banana trees, and coconuts cannot grow, or at least they cannot grow healthy here unless they are kept in a carefully controlled environment. Tropical and subtropical trees cannot thrive in a temperate climate because they wouldn't have the elements needed to sustain their growth.

If I live in a temperate climate like New York State, and I eat food that comes from a tropical environment like Costa Rica, it does something to my internal system. It can throw me, and my endocrine system, out of balance. Eating foods from all over the world sends mixed messages to the pineal gland and to our entire endocrine systems about where we are. Because of these mixed messages, I highly recommend eating locally and seasonally grown food as often as possible. It helps your internal environment (the body's organs and systems) get in harmony with your external environment (where you live), creating a more balanced condition. Eating food that grows in the area where you live can help create and sustain a more harmonious ecosystem for you and for the planet.

If you are a little confused, let's take a closer look at how eating foods grown outside of your climate can negatively affect your endocrine system and your thyroid.

Your pineal gland is the pea-sized gland that sits in the center of your brain. It lives on the endocrine system and is considered your Global Positioning System (GPS) or internal compass, and it controls your body's clock, too. The pineal gland takes in sunlight, temperature, and environmental factors, and regulates your body's circadian rhythms.

The circadian rhythm is responsible for sleeping and waking patterns, endocrine functions, hormone production, digestion and regulation of nutrition, cell regeneration, and many other processes in the body. Disruption of the circadian rhythm leads to insomnia, impaired glucose absorption, diabetes, heart disease, cancer, obesity, depression, and decreased life expectancy.[69]

Regulation of your circadian rhythm requires having access to sunlight and moonlight and eating foods from your environment. Plants require light to grow. The amount of light the plants are exposed to regulates the amount of carbohydrates and sugars the plant contains. When you eat plants, you are eating transmuted sunlight. If you are living in one type of environment/climate and are eating foods from an entirely different environment/climate, your body is receiving mixed messages about where it is. This can disrupt the timing and flow of the natural circadian rhythms in the body.

For purposes of healing the thyroid, it's imperative to get your internal environment aligned with your external environment. You can reset the body's natural circadian rhythms and get into a more harmonious flow by getting outside into nature as often as possible and by eating the foods that are local and seasonal to your environment and ecosystem.

When the body is in harmony and balanced, energy levels naturally increase, including the body's ability to heal. When the body is out of balance, healing may not happen, or it may take a longer time, like in the case of chronic infections that can drain adrenal energy. We have to learn how to work with nature and the environment, not against it.

I had a client from Canada who was suffering from hypothyroidism, and she was freezing all the time. No matter what she

---

69   http://www.nigms.nih.gov/Education/Pages/Factsheet_CircadianRhythms.aspx

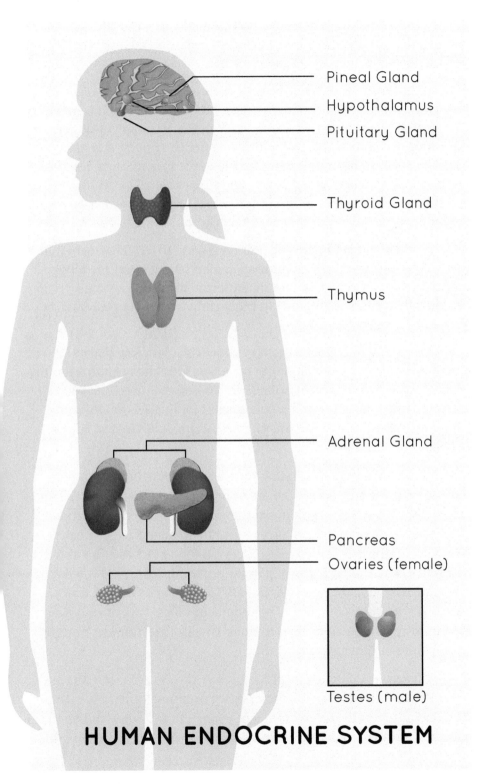

Pineal Gland
Hypothalamus
Pituitary Gland

Thyroid Gland

Thymus

Adrenal Gland

Pancreas
Ovaries (female)

Testes (male)

HUMAN ENDOCRINE SYSTEM

did, she just couldn't warm up her body. When I asked Suzanne about her diet, she told me she was eating lots of fruits and salads every day because she knew they were "good" for her.

Most fruits and salads, by their nature and according to where they grow, are generally cooling. Those foods grow in a much warmer climate than the one she was living in. With every cooling meal she was eating, Suzanne was actually throwing her body more and more out of balance. To heal her condition, she needed warming bone stocks, more animal proteins, saturated fats, and some vegetables heartier than cucumbers and tomatoes. Within a few weeks after altering her diet, Suzanne finally began warming up after years of feeling frozen.

Now, don't get me wrong, I'm not saying to NEVER eat anything that grows outside of your environment. I am saying to eat the foods that can grow within your environment *most often*. You can still occasionally eat food that grows in other climates besides your own, but always let it depend on how you're feeling physically.

For those of you who do NOT know what grows in your environment, you are not alone. As I mentioned in the beginning of this chapter, we are disconnected from Earth. To get reconnected to what's growing in your area, I would highly suggest joining a Community Supported Agriculture (CSA). I talk about this in *Health is Wealth, Make a Delicious Investment in You.*

A CSA is a food-purchasing system where you buy your food directly from the farmers in your area. For example: I pay my farmer and her family $500 in the beginning of the year, and she gives me produce every week for six months. It comes to approximately $21 per week. It is, hands down, the best way to save money on food purchases. It's also the best way to know what is growing in the environment where you live. The farmers in your area cannot *naturally* grow something that is not in harmony with their climate and environment unless they are growing food in temperature-controlled environments like greenhouses or using hydroponics or other means.

I've been a member of a CSA for over two decades, and I have never EVER received a banana or a coconut from my local farmer. Those foods cannot grow in the environment where I live. Understanding that concept, I eat them only occasionally. Certainly not daily in a smoothie!

Regardless of what the marketing and agricultural industries say about the health benefits of bananas or coconut water or any other food that is being marketed to the masses, I know the truth. Those plants simply do not grow anywhere near where my physical body lives. So they are not a part of my daily diet.

There was a young student who attended one of my live cooking classes in New York City. The topic was adrenal health; she attended because she was feeling wiped out. When I began talking about eating local and seasonal foods to balance the body and increase energy, she had a big "aha" moment. She said, "Last year, I began using coconut water and bananas every morning in my smoothie. Initially I felt great, but for the past few months I have been more exhausted than ever. Now I understand why!"

For those of you who don't have access to Community Supported Agriculture, go to a local farmers market to discover what is growing at each specific time of the year in the environment where you live. In the resources section of this book, I've shared with you various websites to help you find farmers and food that grows near you.

Local and seasonal eating is one of the best ways to support your physical body and help get you grounded back to Earth and her frequencies for healing. The food that is growing in the earth picks up the healing vibrations I spoke about in the beginning of this chapter. Every time you eat something that is grown in the earth, rather than in a laboratory, think about that old Beach Boys tune, "Good, good, good, good vibrations!" You are eating those good vibrations, and it'll resonate on the inside of your body.

Speaking of eating, it's time to look at our food—yay! But, before we set the table to sit and eat, we've got to understand some of the healthful foods and healthful habits that may have knocked the thyroid out of balance in the first place. You may be surprised to discover some of the food habits you have been strictly adhering to may be the very things that have promoted your thyroid disease.

CHAPTER 8
Healthful Food Habits That Are Not So Healthful

I hear from frustrated *"healthy"* eaters all the time. They complain, "I am eating the healthiest foods in the world and I can't lose weight! Why isn't my thyroid working? It just doesn't make any sense!"

Actually, it makes a *lot* of sense. This is one of the biggest obstacles to healing the thyroid, because much of what we have been taught about healthful foods throughout the past few decades may, in fact, be quite the opposite of what our bodies need. The health-related information that has been shoved down our throats may be downright harmful to our health.

Not all healthful foods or eating habits are good for all people. So, before you swallow a billion probiotics or reach for the vegetable crudités and nonfat dip at the next party, you may want to continue reading.

THE FAT FACTS

Many health-conscious folks have severely restricted, or completely eliminated, saturated fat from their diets, usually for weight-loss and heart health. I was one of these people. I spent a lifetime counting fat grams, deathly afraid of eating fat for fear it would make me fat, or worse yet, give me a heart attack!

I peeled the crispy skin off Roasted Rosemary Chicken and discarded it as the "bad-for-me" part of the meal. Sometimes I'd guiltily sneak a bite or two before tossing it into the garbage. And, man-oh-man, was that little piece of skin heavenly! Simply licking the chicken fat off my fingers was deeply satisfying.

I was also one of those annoying people always asking for "dressing on the side." And, I certainly wouldn't allow any savory gravy to moisten my holiday turkey. Heck no! "I'll have mine plain, white meat only, please." The white meat had less fat and, interestingly, less flavor and moisture as well. I would smother that dry turkey breast with a cup of sugary cranberry sauce to help moisten it and make it easier to swallow.

Egg white omelets cooked in olive oil were another staple for me. And, I wouldn't even dare think about buttering my whole grain toast, "I'll take mine dry as cardboard, please."

Besides depriving my palate of the luscious flavor of fat, I was simultaneously depriving my body of essential vitamins and minerals. Vitamins A, D, E, K, and B12 are all fat-soluble. These vitamins are usually absorbed in fat globules (called chylomicrons) that travel through the lymphatic system of the small intestines and into the general blood circulation within the body. These fat-soluble vitamins, especially vitamins A and E, are then stored in body tissues.[70]

Vitamins A and D are required for protein and calcium assimilation, to create hormones, and support the endocrine system. Low levels of vitamin D are associated with autoimmune diseases including multiple sclerosis, rheumatoid arthritis, thyroiditis, and Crohn's disease.[71]

Some of the best sources of vitamins A and D are found in animal proteins and saturated animal fats: fish, shellfish, fish liver, eggs, organ meats, butter, cream, and other saturated fats.[72] Unfortunately, these are the very same foods that have been demonized by many health advocates, including me when I was vegetarian-turned-vegan in my early thirties. Thankfully, with age comes wisdom and I now butter my toast, eat the whole egg with the yolk, and enjoy crispy chicken skin—without any guilt.

A low-fat or no-fat diet or a diet high in the wrong type of fat weakens immunity and contributes to poor healing and a malfunctioning hormonal system.[73] Our unnatural fear of fat is especially harmful to the adrenals and the thyroid. Fat is necessary for energy and maintaining cell integrity and hormone production. The hormones in our bodies are derived from cholesterol and lipids (fat).

What I've discovered in my health-coaching practice is that when people, especially women, don't eat fat, they actually crave more sugar and carbohydrates. Those excess carbohydrates are converted into sugar, and eventually converted once again and stored as—yep, you guessed it—FAT! Trust me, you are better off eating good quality saturated fat than sugar and excess carbohydrates that eventually turn to fat.

---

70 http://www.medicinenet.com/script/main/art.asp?articlekey=10736
71 http://www.westonaprice.org/basicnutrition/vitamindmiracle.html#food
72 Eat Fat, Lose Fat, By Dr. Mary Enig & Sally Fallon, Penguin Group 2004, pg. 50-54
73 Overcoming Thyroid Disorders, David Brownstein M.D., Medical Alternative Press, 2008, pg. 242

Time and time again when clients get permission to eat fat, they usually discover a change in mood. Within one week of incorporating saturated fats into their diets, many clients tell me they don't know why but they suddenly feel happier, are less likely to snack and binge on sweets, and are more satisfied overall.

Fat satisfies us on a deep level. "When we eat real cholesterol and fat, we regulate insulin levels and trigger enzymes that convert food into energy. Cholesterol from food modulates our body's internal cholesterol production and protects liver function."[74]

For the sake of your thyroid, endocrine system, and liver, eat some good old-fashioned saturated fat derived from animal products. And, of course continue eating monounsaturated fats like olive oil and polyunsaturated fats like nut and seed oils, but not in excess. Vegetable and other plant-based fats (nut and seed oils) in excess can contribute to higher rates of inflammation.[75]

The fats to completely steer clear of are the fake fats. These are the fats created from vegetable oils that are designed to look, taste, and feel like saturated animal fats. These include hydrogenated fats like margarine, vegetable shortenings, and the so-called healthful butter substitutes you find in every health food store and supermarket. Do NOT eat these fats. Not even on a dare. These particular fats have wreaked havoc on our health. "They adversely affect our cholesterol levels by increasing LDL and lowering HDL, and they interfere with insulin production, promoting diabetes and obesity."[76]

Make no mistake about it, faux fat makes you FAT and unhealthy! "In the Nurse's Health Study, women who consumed the greatest amount of trans fats (in the form of hydrogenated oil) in their diet had a 50 percent higher risk of heart attack than women who consumed the least."[77]

Eat real fat, the kind your ancestors ate. They were strong hearty people and weren't dropping dead of heart attacks and strokes; mostly, this is a modern phenomenon.

74   http://www.womentowomen.com/healthyweight/fatandcholesterol.aspx
75   http://chriskresser.com/how-too-much-omega-6-and-not-enough-omega-3-is-making-us-sick
76   fat: An appreciation of a misunderstood ingredient, By Jennifer McLagan, Ten Speed Press, 2008, pg. 9
77   http://www.webmd.com/diet/features/trans-fats-science-and-risks?page=2

Some of the best and most easily absorbable sources of saturated fat, which contain vitamins A and D, are found in many of the foods that have been labeled unhealthful. These foods include whole eggs, organ meats like liver, and grass-fed butter.[78] Current studies confirm these formerly unhealthful foods are actually pretty darn healthful for us, so don't be afraid to put a little pat of butter on your steamed vegetables and let it nourish you on a deeper level.

SUGAR SUBSTITUTES

We all know sugar, in large quantities, is bad for our health. This is probably the one indisputable fact that all scientists, food advocates, and health seekers agree upon. But, here's where the trouble begins. To wean us off our addiction to sugar, many food scientists, dieticians, and diet-oriented folks have encouraged artificial sweeteners as more healthful sugar substitutes. Don't fall for this delusion!

For the sake of your thyroid, and the rest of your beautiful body, eliminate ALL artificial sweeteners from your diet: sucralose, Splenda, saccharin, stevia, Nuva, Truvia, aspartame, NutraSweet, Equal, and any others. The manufacturers of food keep coming out with new sugar substitutes on a yearly basis. By the time you read this book, there may already be fifty new sugar substitutes on the market. All of these faux sugars are not better for us. In fact, they can be much much worse for us.

From a chef's perspective, artificial sweeteners leave an odd aftertaste on the tongue. Artificial sweeteners also have a sweeter flavor profile than sugar, some of them being fifteen to three hundred times sweeter than sugar! That extreme sweet flavor can damage your delicate palate.

We all have taste receptors in our mouth: sweet, sour, salty, bitter, pungent/spicy, and umami (savory). If we oversweet ourselves by eating something ten times sweeter than sugar, it can inhibit our ability to taste sweetness in food provided for us by the natural environment. When your palate is overwhelmed by extremely sweet sugar substitutes, a crisp sweet apple or fresh juicy berries lose their naturally sweet appeal.

Besides the flavor factor, chemical sweeteners are downright dangerous to our health! Check out these facts about aspartame (Nutrasweet, Equal) that is found in almost every food product from gum to yogurt, including many sugar-free foods for children.

78   http://www.huffingtonpost.com/christiane-northrup/saturated-fat_b_4914235.html

"Aspartame is made up of aspartic acid, phenylalanine, and methanol. Aspartame changes the ratio of amino acids in the blood, blocking or lowering the levels of serotonin, tyrosine, dopamine, norepinephrine, and adrenaline.[79] Blocking and lowering our hormones screws up the physical body, especially the endocrine system.

An interesting phenomenon that many clients experience once they stop ingesting diet soda and diet food laced with chemical sweeteners is that they naturally begin losing weight and their headaches and other bodily aches begin to disappear. Coincidence? No, it's just common sense. When we put chemicals into our body that disrupt our perfectly designed hormonal system, we feel the effects all the way down to our bones.

You are better off using small amounts of natural sugars, like local raw honey, maple syrup, beet and cane sugars, than chemical and artificial sweeteners any day of the week.

OY! SO MUCH SOY!

Traditionally fermented soy can be quite healthful for many people and has been a staple food in many Asian cultures. These health-promoting products include tempeh, miso, shoyu, natto, tofu, and tamari.

In America we've mass-produced soybeans without properly fermenting them to release the antinutrients, goitrogens, and enzyme inhibitors they contain. Soybeans that aren't properly processed through traditional sprouting and fermenting methods have been linked to thyroid disease, digestive problems, reproductive disorders, infertility, cancer, and other illnesses.[80] [81]

Healthy folks in the know already understand that unfermented soy foods can be problematic for the thyroid and can promote a goiter. These foods include soy milk, soy meats, soy nuts, soy chips, soy yogurt, soy ice cream, and many other unfermented soy products.[82]

What many people do NOT realize is that they may be eating unfermented, nontraditional soy ingredients and not even know it. Soy can be disguised as isolated soy protein, textured vegetable

---

79   http://www.sweetpoison.com/aspartame-side-effects.html
80   http://www.scientificamerican.com/article/soybean-fertility-hormone-isoflavones-genistein/
81   http://articles.mercola.com/sites/articles/archive/2010/10/13/soy-controversy-and-health-effects.aspx
82   http://www.doctoroz.com/videos/soy-good-bad-and-best?page=2

protein, hydrolyzed vegetable protein, lecithin, bouillon, natural flavors, monosodium glutamate (MSG), mono- and diglycerides, and plant protein.[83]

Soy has saturated our food supply! Those energy bars, natural snack bars, protein powders, and healthful breakfast cereals may contain highly processed soy ingredients that could be damaging the digestive system and thyroid.

No matter how healthful a food claims to be, read the label and check the ingredients. You may be surprised to discover you are eating nonfermented soy more often than you think.

A STRICT VEGAN DIET

Many health-obsessed people, at some point in their lives, adopt a vegan diet. That may be a pretty good idea because we are overeating meat and not eating enough plants. Too often, unfortunately, I've witnessed students and clients who have taken on strict vegan diets suffer from nutritional deficiencies, pernicious anemia, adrenal fatigue, and thyroid disease.

"One of the many results of lack of protein is hypothyroidism because animal protein is required to make the thyroid hormone and to convert it to its active form in the liver."[84]

I get emails almost every day from vegans telling me that they've read my blog or one of my books, and they want to know good sources of absorbable plant-based protein because they refuse to eat meat. My advice to them is that I do not recommend veganism for healing the thyroid or the adrenals. I tell them to continue eating plants because they are really good for health, and to *supplement* their diet with naturally raised animal proteins because they are good for health, too.

A young lady, in her late twenties, came for health coaching. Jennifer was suffering from hair loss and an underactive thyroid. She was much too young to be losing her hair. She said it was coming out in clumps, and the hair that did remain on her head was breaking and splitting. I asked when the hair loss began, and she told me about eight months prior. She also told me she had transitioned to a raw vegan diet about one and a half years earlier.

83   http://articles.mercola.com/sites/articles/archive/2011/12/08/the-dirty-little-secret-hidden-in-much-of-your-health-food.aspx
84   Thyroid Resistance By Lita Lee, Ph.D.

I advised that maybe it was time to reconsider her raw vegan diet and start eating some cooked foods and animal proteins, and she cried, "I can't eat meat! If I eat meat, I am going to die from cancer! All of the books I've read told me that eating meat is carcinogenic and bad for me. I don't want to die from cancer."

I said, "I understand your situation. At one point in my life, I was vegan too. It's a fantastic way to cleanse the body, and it certainly gave me greater reverence for animals and how they are raised and treated. In the beginning of my vegan journey, I felt fantastic, but within a year, I didn't feel so well any more. For the sake of my health, I had to reevaluate my diet. A vegan way of eating doesn't work for everyone and can lead to deficiencies in some people."

Jennifer cried even harder, "That can't possibly be true! All of the books I've read couldn't *all* be wrong about the same thing."

As I was listening to her, I was reminded of a funny quote from Mark Twain. He said, "Be careful about reading health books. You may die of a misprint."

Always check in with your physical body to see if the food you are eating is actually working for you. I remind clients and students to question *everything*, and that includes *everything* I say. Take the information you read in any book, including this one, and apply it to your own physical body. Let your body be the judge. Do you feel healthy and vibrant? If yes, continue what you're doing. If not, it's time to make some changes.

PALEO, PRIMAL, AND CRO-MAGNON DIETS

Returning to our caveman roots is all the rage. And, it can work like a charm to help get excess weight off the body. I remember when I was suffering from candida overgrowth, I took almost ALL the carbs out of my diet and ate mostly protein and vegetables. Wow! I lost a lot of weight. I went down to 118 pounds. But, within a few months of my high protein, no-carb/low-carb diet, I began feeling a constricted and tight sensation throughout my body. My candida was in check, but I was too skinny, wasn't feeling vibrant or healthy, and my energy was crashing. I knew this dietary approach wasn't balanced in dealing with candida, and it was affecting my thyroid as well. You can read more about healing candida on my website **www.AndreaBeaman.com**.

I've also worked with many clients who took on a paleo-type diet and they developed hypothyroid conditions. This can happen for a couple of reasons. Firstly, insulin is needed for the conversion of T4 to T3, and insulin is generally low on a paleo diet. Secondly, cortisol can increase on a high-protein low-carbohydrate diet, and when that happens, your adrenals become stressed, which naturally slows the thyroid.[85]

I've met many folks who felt AMAZING at the beginning of a new eating regimen, but within a few years, they didn't feel so well anymore—even though they hadn't changed the regimen. Always keep in mind that a food plan may work for a while and then may stop working for various reasons. Be open to changing and growing when that happens.

THE RAW REVOLUTION

Many plants contain antinutrients that can inhibit thyroid function. The Brassicaceae (cruciferous) family of vegetables contains glucosinolates that can inhibit iodine uptake, resulting in hypothyroidism and promoting goiter formation.[86] This family of plants includes some of the most noble and celebrated vegetables including kale, broccoli, cauliflower, cabbage, and Brussels sprouts.

If you are currently suffering from hypothyroidism, goiter, or any other form of thyroid disease, I suggest you steer clear of the raw cruciferous vegetable platter and kale juice for a while because eating them may be a recipe for disaster!

Now, this doesn't mean you need to completely avoid these powerhouse veggies; just make sure they are prepared properly. Cooking with heat and salt can help deactivate some of their goitrogenic properties, and eating an iodine-rich diet can help as well.

Funnily enough, I often hear from people suffering from hyperthyroidism who tell me they have incorporated raw cruciferous vegetables into their diets because they have read that these vegetables inhibit the uptake of iodine and stop the thyroid from functioning. What these folks don't understand is that even people suffering from hyperthyroidism, Hashimoto's, or Graves' need iodine. The problem is that those people are not absorbing the iodine properly. Every cell in our body needs iodine to function. Not only does eating raw cruciferous

85   http://chriskresser.com/is-a-low-carb-diet-ruining-your-health/
86   http://lpi.oregonstate.edu/infocenter/foods/cruciferous/

veggies NOT heal folks suffering from hyperthyroidism and Graves', but it can actually make the problem worse. Too many raw cold foods, in general, can lead to a cold digestive system resulting in malabsorption of nutrients, which can lead to anemia. I personally LOVE raw veggies, especially when I'm cleansing in the spring or I need to cool down on a hot summer day. But, the raw veggies I eat are generally not from the Brassicacae family. Instead I eat light salad greens (lettuces), cucumbers, sprouts, and herbs. In the recipe section, you have a variety of both raw and cooked foods to choose from.

SMOOTHIE CENTRAL

Smoothies are quick and easy and smooth and creamy. Every health fanatic is drinking them: green smoothies, fruit smoothies, protein smoothies, breakfast smoothies, maca smoothies, cacao smoothies. Holy cacao! We've gone smoothie crazy! BUT, smoothies can actually damage the digestive system and weaken the body in the long term. Many smoothies contain frozen fruit and fresh or frozen greens plus some type of milky substance like almond milk, soy milk, coconut milk, rice milk, or dairy milk. This can be a triple whammy for the thyroid!

First off, many of those smoothies contain raw greens like kale or raw green powders that contain goitrogenic vegetables. As mentioned, goitrogens are substances that can inhibit the body's ability to use iodine, promote goiter formation, and act like antithyroid drugs, causing hypothyroidism.

Secondly, if that smoothie contains coconut milk, soy milk, rice milk, or almond milk, it may also contain carrageenan, which is a common ingredient in those milks. Carrageenan is a controversial ingredient that has been linked with cancer, inflammation, and digestive distress.[87] Many thyroid conditions, especially autoimmune conditions like Hashimoto's and Graves', stem from poor gut health and digestive problems.[88]

Thirdly, humans are not designed to drink carbohydrates and proteins. Our food needs to be partially broken down by the process of chewing and by the chemical action of being mixed with salivary enzymes. If our food isn't mixed with saliva to start the process of digestion, we can suffer from a whole host of tummy troubles.

Food, even though it may be liquefied, still needs to be mixed with the enzymes in saliva to be digested. If you are drinking smoothies,

---

87   http://chriskresser.com/harmful-or-harmless-carrageenan
88   http://www.ncbi.nlm.nih.gov/pmc/articles/PMC2699000/

you are gulping down carbohydrates, gulping down proteins, gulping down sugars, and setting yourself up for digestive distress and strain on the pancreas. If you bypass the digestive enzymes in the mouth, the pancreas has to do double the work.

My husband occasionally likes using those green powders and protein powders. When I was thinking about what to tell you about those smoothie-enhancing products, I actually read the ingredients on my hubby's *super green powder*. It contained *everything* you don't actually want to eat RAW, plus raw yucca root.

Yucca root contains saponins that can be toxic to humans, especially when eaten raw. Yucca was traditionally pounded and then fried or boiled. Yucca is a tropical root and was prepared the way people eat other starchy roots or tubers like potatoes—COOKED!

Many people are also drinking smoothies with raw maca root. Raw maca is a powerful goitrogen that can inhibit thyroid function as well. Native people from South America never ate maca raw. It was always fermented and cooked before being eaten.

Of course, we also have the super-duper "healthy" folks who put raw cacao nibs into their smoothies. This is a BIG no-no for thyroid health. Raw cacao has theobromine and mycotoxins that can overstimulate the heart, mind, and nervous system. Overstimulation can eventually lead to burnout and adrenal fatigue.

I often hear from health coaches and health advocates who tell me they are adding raw cacao nibs and raw maca root to their green smoothies. They don't understand why they can't sleep at night or why they are having heart palpitations and anxiety or why they've been diagnosed with thyroid disease.

Just because something is marketed and advertised as a super food does not mean it necessarily is, nor does it mean that it is good for you. A good rule of thumb is to look at how traditional and native peoples ate and drank these foods. Beyond the phytonutrients and antioxidants and the scientific knowledge that we have today, native peoples were much wiser than we are when it came to preparation of food. They listened to their physical bodies and were intuitively connected to the plants they were eating.

This does not mean you can *never* have a smoothie again. I'm not the anti-smoothie girl! Smoothies are fun. They can also help lighten the digestive load, especially when you're cleansing. Just don't have smoothies on a daily basis. And, remember to swish them around your mouth and combine them with your saliva before swallowing.

I would recommend that while you are healing your digestive system and your thyroid, you have smoothies infrequently, maybe one or two times per week. And, do NOT have frozen smoothies for breakfast! Egads! Cold food in the morning is not a good idea when you are trying to heal the digestive system and support the thyroid.

Breakfast means to "break the fast." When we sleep at night, we are fasting (not eating food), and we are not consciously moving our muscles. This causes our bodies' temperature to lower. In the morning, it's always been best to break the fast with something warm.

Eating something ice cold like a frozen smoothie or boxed breakfast cereal with cold milk requires extra effort from the body to stoke the digestive fire. Consistently eating iced or cold food in the morning can exhaust energy reserves and inhibit the process of digestion for the entire day.

Many cultures around the world traditionally eat something warm in the morning. Some people eat soft porridge or some type of gruel for breakfast. Others eat a variety of soups or congees that were made from cooked rice, corn, rye, or other grains combined with water, animal milk, or coconut milk. Heartier breakfasts included eggs, bacon, sausages, and bread with butter. In the past one hundred years, we have radically altered that traditional warm breakfast and now begin the day with the exact opposite: frozen smoothies and hard cereals with ice-cold milk. Not smart!

The type of breakfast we choose can either support us in starting our day or make us want to crawl right back into bed. I alternate my breakfasts. Some days I'll have a poached egg on kasha pilaf, or scrambled eggs with sourdough toast and butter. Other days, it's oatmeal with nuts, seeds, and berries with a little bit of yogurt, kefir, or cream on top. Sometimes I'll have miso soup with mochi (pounded sweet rice) or leftover rice. I also love eggs on top of root hash, or a frittata with a side salad. You get the picture?

Vary your breakfast choices depending on the season and how you're physically feeling on any particular day. There are a lot of great breakfast options, and I've included them in the recipe section. Experiment with your body, and see what type of food makes you feel best.

ONE BILLION PROBIOTICS

One of my clients who took probiotic capsules complained about feeling gassy and bloated all the time. Because these symptoms can be indicators of decreased liver function as well as bacterial overgrowth, I suggested she stop taking probiotic capsules and instead incorporate some bug-killing herbs for a while. I advised that she take an herbal supplement containing black walnut hull, wormwood, quassia bark, garlic, plus oregano oil. You can find something similar to this at your local health food store, or you can buy individual herbal tinctures and follow the instructions on the labels.

Within two weeks, the bloating she had suffered from for almost two years disappeared. Now she swears that her bloating and gas began when she first started taking probiotic capsules. And, she may be right. As long as rogue bacteria are populating the digestive system, they are going to EAT the probiotics you send them, and they are going to thrive.

Over 70 percent of our immunity lives in the gut. If the digestive system is overrun by rogue bacteria and viruses, immunity can become compromised.

The first thing I like to do with clients suffering from autoimmune thyroid conditions, or any thyroid conditions, is to clean up their internal environments: their digestive systems and their diets. That starts with their getting off the processed junk, sugar, artificial sweeteners, excessive carbohydrates, and any extreme dieting behavior (paleo, veganism, smoothie-ism), and getting the rogue bacteria in check by doing a bug-killing and deworming protocol. Then these folks begin eating a wholesome, balanced natural-foods diet, including probiotic-rich foods like sauerkraut, kimchi, pickles, yogurt, and kefir. I do not recommend powdered probiotic products that contain extremely high doses of bacteria. The physical body may not need, or be able to handle, fifty billion microorganisms (or more) in one shot, the dosage of many probiotics. Another thought for you to digest is that when probiotic bacteria enter the body in the form of food, it is processed differently, more organically, so to speak.

Speaking of food, it's time for you to learn about what types of foods to eat and how to prepare them to help support your digestive system and start healing your condition. With knowledge comes power, so let's get to know some of the fabulous foods that can benefit the health of your thyroid!

CHAPTER 9
Thyroid-Nourishing Foods

Knowing what to eat should be a simple and pleasurable experience, but for many folks, food choice can create quite a panic! Especially, when it comes to healing thyroid conditions.

As you've read in the previous chapter, there is a lot of nutritional nonsense that the experts have given us throughout the years, but what they haven't given us is any knowledge about the traditional preparation of food. This is where the trouble lies. If you are eating improperly prepared foods, you could be damaging your health.

WHOLE GRAINS

For thousands of years, grains have been eaten by many of the world's populations. The difference between the whole grains our ancestors ate and the refined grains we eat today is vast; many of the refined grains have lost most of their vital elements during the milling process and are nutritionally deficient. To make up for this deficiency, bread and cereal manufacturers began to "fortify" many of their products with vitamins and minerals.

Additionally, the starches in highly refined grains are absorbed quickly, spiking blood sugar levels. Blood sugar instability contributes to type II diabetes, obesity, inflammation, insulin resistance, and heart disease.[89]

On the other hand, traditional whole grains can contribute to a good night's sleep, create a balanced feeling in the body, satisfy hunger, and promote smooth bowel movements, long memory, and clear thinking. According to author Steve Gagne, "Energetically, whole cereal grains finely tune the human nervous system in such a way as to affect every part of the body, to the extent of unifying it with the soul as one whole functioning organism. This was the legacy given us by our ancestors."[90]

Whole cereal grains are carbohydrates. I've worked with many clients who were suffering from brain fog and an inability to think clearly from abusing carbohydrates, and that includes whole grains. I've also worked with folks who have gone completely grain free, and

89   http://www.scientificamerican.com/article/carbs-against-cardio/
90   The Energetics of Food, Steve Gagne, 2006, pg. 295

they discovered that going without grains did NOT heal their thyroid conditions, and in many cases, had made them feel worse. We need carbohydrates for energy production, and to convert thyroid hormones.

What is true is that not ALL grains work for ALL people, and ALL grains need to be prepared properly to benefit health. Whole grains were traditionally prepared by soaking, sprouting, fermenting, and cooking. This process made them more digestible and increased nutritional potency.

By rushing to produce food for the mass market, many of our traditional preparation techniques have been lost. All grains (beans, nuts, and seeds, too) contain phytic acid, antinutrient compounds that reduce the body's ability to absorb nutrients, and enzyme inhibitors that exist in the outer layer of the bran. Phytic acid can bind with calcium, magnesium, copper, iron, and especially zinc, and block their absorption. Zinc supports thyroid function because it is required to convert thyroid hormones T4 to T3, and iron is critical for building strong blood. Many thyroid patients suffer from anemia (low blood iron). Magnesium is crucial for relaxing the muscles and helps thyroid patients, both men and women, who often complain of muscle cramping, especially in the middle of the night when they are trying to get some sleep!

Refining the grain by stripping the outer bran eliminates the potential phytic acid problem, but also eliminates essential nutrients, bran, and fiber. Before eating any whole grains, it's best to use traditional preparation methods. Soaking grain is one of those methods that releases 40 to 70 percent of antinutrients. Grains that have already been heat treated, like rolled oats and kasha, do not need to be soaked before cooking.

Cooking deactivates many antinutrients in the grain, which is one of the reasons I do NOT recommend eating raw sprouted grains. The preparation process is simply not complete without roasting or cooking. There are many foods you can eat raw, but not whole grains.

Our ancestors cooked their grains. Let's follow their lead. They intuitively knew better than modern nutritional science and dietary fads about what to eat and how to prepare it. Some appropriate grains for healing a thyroid condition can include brown rice, quinoa, kasha, oats, polenta, and wild rice. Heartier grains containing gluten, like wheat, barley, and rye, can be difficult to digest, especially, if they are not properly prepared or if you have an underlying digestive issue or autoimmune condition.

When people from thyroid communities discover that I eat gluten-containing grains, they usually respond with, "Andrea, you of all people, should know better! Don't you know how BAD gluten is for you?"

It seems whenever some new concept takes hold of the masses, we are all supposed to fall in line without question. That's not the way I roll. I question everything. Regardless of what anyone tells me, or what the "ever-changing science" surrounding the newest food fad says, I always research the traditional ways people ate specific foods, and then experiment with them to discover the effects on my own body.

For centuries, Asians ate wheat-based noodles; the French ate croissants; people in the Middle-East ate chapatis and pita bread; and all over Europe, various types of bread have been staple foods. Wheat was even called the "staff of life" by the ancient Egyptians.

So, what happened to wheat and other glutinous products to deserve such a bad rap? The first reason is obvious: the human digestive system has deteriorated due to the consumption of large amounts of sugar, highly processed and chemical-laden foods, excess stress, lack of chewing, moms' not breastfeeding their babies, and the overuse of antibiotics, which destroys intestinal flora. But, it's much easier to blame the wheat and gluten for our sudden onslaught of digestive woes.

As a species, we are destroying our intestinal fortitude. If our digestive system is weak, we simply will NOT be able to process food properly, no matter what it is.

The second reason is that modern wheat was hybridized to contain higher levels of gluten that could withstand the mechanized process of commercial production of mass quantities of bread in the shortest amount of time.[91] Hybridized wheat can be problematic because it contains higher levels of gluten than traditional varieties of wheat.

For thousands of years, humans took time to prepare glutinous grains by using a process that required patience; it was called fermentation. Ancient bakers used sourdough starter that contained wild yeast and several strains of lactobacilli. And, we all know how beneficial lactobacilli can be for a hungry digestive system! Lactobacilli

---

91   http://www.westonaprice.org/modern-diseases/against-the-grain/

are the friendly bacteria that normally live in our digestive, urinary, and genital systems and help us digest food, absorb nutrients, and fight off unfriendly disease-promoting bacteria.[92]

Interestingly, recent studies by Italian scientists have shown that traditionally prepared sourdough bread had NO negative effects on the digestive tract of those suffering from celiac disease.[93]

For those of you who don't understand the science behind this amazing phenomenon, it's as simple as this: traditionally processed sourdough bread made with bacterial starter breaks down gluten proteins, making it easier to digest and more beneficial for us.[94] [95]

A fluffy loaf of naturally leavened sourdough contains flour, water, salt, starter, and time. That's it!

Many people suffering from thyroid disease have taken gluten OUT of their diets and have put gluten-free substitutes in. This is a bad idea. I cringe reading the long list of ingredients on some of those gluten-free breads and other gluten-free products. Egads! If you don't already have a digestive problem you are surely going to give yourself one. Sorghum, contained in many gluten-free products can be extremely hard to digest, especially if not processed properly. Tapioca starch and almond flour, in large quantities on a daily basis, can lead to inflammation and thyroid troubles. And, xanthan gum, used in many gluten-free products, can cause gastrointestinal distress, lung problems, and blood sugar imbalances.[96]

Don't get me wrong. Sourdough bread and other gluten containing products are NOT good for everyone, nor do I think they are BAD for everyone.

I personally couldn't imagine life without Poached Eggs on Sourdough Toast that is slathered in grass-fed butter. It's one of my favorite breakfasts. Dunking that crispy sourdough bread into a gooey egg yolk... oh my! It's a mouthful of bliss.

But, while you are healing any autoimmune thyroid condition or digestive issue, it would be wise to remove gluten grains from your diet for

92   http://www.nlm.nih.gov/medlineplus/druginfo/natural/790.html
93   http://www.cghjournal.org/article/S1542-3565(10)00987-0/abstract
94   http://www.ncbi.nlm.nih.gov/pmc/articles/PMC348803/
95   http://fyiliving.com/diet/special-diets/allergies-food-sensitivities/celiacs-can-say-yes-to-sourdough-bread/
96   http://www.webmd.com/vitamins-supplements/ingredientmono-340-XANTHAN%20GUM.aspx?activeIngredientId=340&activeIngredientName=XANTHAN%20GUM

a period of time (three months to two years) to help heal your condition. But, the good news is, you may not have to take them out forever.

BEANS & LEGUMES

Beans and grains naturally complement each other and have traditionally been served together. For example, rice and black beans are a staple in many Latin cultures as are hummus (chickpeas) and pita bread in Middle Eastern cuisine, dal (lentils) and naan bread in India, black beans and corn tortillas in the Americas, pasta e fagioli (bean and pasta soup) in Italy. Red beans and rice is a famous New Orleans dish here in the United States.

Many cultures often paired beans with some type of fat as well. This pairing enhances flavor, nutrition, and digestibility. Beans contain protein and carbohydrates. If you count the carbohydrate content in beans, it by far surpasses the protein. Combining beans with fat helps slow the absorption of carbohydrates, keeping blood sugar balanced.

Some traditional bean and fat combinations include hummus, which contains the oil of sesame seeds (tahini), traditional cassoulet from France prepared with duck or goose fat, and in Mexico, Latin countries, and the Mediterranean, beans were combined with lard, olive oil, or other fat.

I remember growing up in America eating canned baked beans that always came with a small cube of pork fat. We kids would always fight over who got that creamy little mouthwatering lump. Not only did the fat make the beans taste savory and delicious, it also was rich in vitamins A and D, which benefit the endocrine system and bones.

Beans often get a bad rap because folks can have difficulty digesting them.

As mentioned, the digestive system in modern humans has been compromised. With our sorry state of intestinal health, digestion of beans, as well as many other foods, becomes difficult.

Beans need to be properly prepared to make them more digestible. This includes soaking them for eight to twenty-four hours to release acids, antinutrients, gas-causing enzymes, and trisaccharides (sugars).

I highly recommend soaking beans with a small piece of kelp sea vegetable. Kelp contains glutamic acid, which helps to soften tough fibers, making beans more digestible and produce less gas. That'll make your friends and family happy, for sure! Some people suggest adding a tablespoon of vinegar to the soaking water to help neutralize the bean's antinutrients, but I've found that sometimes this keeps the beans hard. That could be a good thing if you are using the beans for a salad and want the beans to retain their shape without falling apart.

Beans take time to prepare, but they are worth it. I personally LOVE beans: chili, burritos, rice and beans, bean soup, hummus with pita or vegetable crudités—yum! Small beans like lentils, adukis, black-eyed peas, and navy beans can be cooked in one hour or less, but larger beans like kidney, garbanzo, and cannellini can take two hours or longer.

The beauty of cooking beans is that you don't have to baby sit them. Put them on the stove with the appropriate amount of water; bring to a boil. Skim and discard the foam that rises to the top. Adjust the temperature to simmer, and cover. No need to stir or sauté—they practically cook themselves.

I understand we're all busy, so if you do not have time to prepare beans from scratch, use canned beans. Keep in mind, though, that many canned foods contain endocrine-disrupting Bisphenol A (BPA) in the hard plastic coating on the inside of the can. BPA disrupts the functioning of the thyroid gland and endocrine system.[97] There are many brands in the marketplace that have BPA-free cans. Look for them.

Something else to keep in mind when eating beans is "quantity changes quality." I had a client who was suffering from Hashimoto's and goiter. We altered her diet, and she started feeling better rather quickly. Within one month, she stopped losing her hair, felt less swollen in her neck, and had sustainable energy levels. BUT, Jennifer noticed whenever she ate hummus, she broke out in a rash on her stomach and became bloated and uncomfortable. To get to the bottom of this gaseous dilemma, I asked her to keep a food journal.

She realized she was eating hummus two and three times per day as a "healthful snack." Plus, because it was a snack and not a meal, she always rushed through eating the hummus and was forgetting to chew. Even though hummus is garbanzo beans that have been pureed into a slurry, it still needs to be mixed with saliva, otherwise it can contribute to digestive distress and bloating. Hummus can easily slide down the

97   http://www.ncbi.nlm.nih.gov/pubmed/23238275

throat without your chewing it. Thank goodness for the pita bread or vegetable crudités that usually accompanies it. When hummus and pita are paired, as it was traditionally eaten, this ensures some amount of chewing.

Not all beans work for thyroid conditions; one of those is soy. Soybeans contain potent enzyme inhibitors and goitrogens that inhibit thyroid function. In many Asian cultures, soybeans were fermented before eating, and that deactivated their negative effects.

Soybeans have been a healthful staple in many Asian cultures because of the way they were prepared and eaten. Some healthful soy products include tempeh, miso, shoyu, natto, tofu, and tamari. These soy foods were generally eaten in small quantities. When you eat miso soup in a Japanese restaurant, you'll notice there are little tiny cubes of tofu, not big chunks.

Sometimes *health-conscious* eaters will overeat something because of its scientifically proven healing benefits, as in the case of soy. Always remember that quantity changes quality. In America, instead of eating small cubes of tofu, we've taken whole blocks of tofu and turned it into faux chicken salad or faux egg salad, and then we eat the entire container. Not healthful! Those soybeans have not been properly processed. Soybeans that aren't properly processed through traditional fermenting methods have been linked to thyroid disease, digestive problems, reproductive disorders, and other troubles.[98]

Some not-so-healthful soy products include isolated soy proteins that are in many of those heavily marketed health or energy bars and protein powders, soy dogs, soy burgers, soy meats, soymilk, soy ice cream, soy yogurts, soy margarine, soy chips, and soy nuts. These highly processed soy foods are "health food junk foods," so don't eat large quantities of them, or don't eat them at all.

I eat fermented soy products like miso soup and I love it! It has wonderful digestive properties, and it's rich in iodine from the added seaweed. I often recommend miso soup with seaweed one to three times per week for people suffering from thyroid cancer, and all other thyroid conditions, too. Just because someone has hyperthyroidism or Hashimoto's does not mean they shouldn't eat iodine-rich foods. The thyroid needs iodine. It just needs the right type of iodine in the right

---

98   http://articles.mercola.com/sites/articles/archive/2010/10/13/soy-controversy-and-health-effects.aspx

quantities. The wrong type of iodine is in all of the processed foods that many folks are eating.

As you can see, beans and legumes of all types can be delicious additions to a thyroid-healthful diet, but you need to become aware of how they are prepared and eaten. I've provided delicious bean recipes for you in the recipe section.

VEGETABLES

I love vegetables! I love them raw, steamed, sautéed, roasted, fermented—you name it, I love it. Vegetables contain a wide spectrum of vitamins, minerals, phytonutrients, and antioxidants.

Unfortunately, the scientific information regarding the importance of vitamins and minerals in vegetables has been exploited. People revere vegetables as if they are the end all of everything. It's not necessarily true.

Eating too many vegetables can ruin your health as quickly as not eating enough vegetables. One of the keys to healing the thyroid is that beyond any phytonutrients, antioxidants, or vitamins and minerals, it's best to eat seasonally and locally grown produce. This can help create a balanced body.

As mentioned in previous chapters, most folks do NOT know what foods are local and seasonal to their environment because everything is available ALL the time. Just because produce is in the grocery store does NOT mean it's the right food for your body. Veggies and fruits can actually damage your digestive terrain, lower vitamin D levels, and throw the endocrine system out of balance when eaten IN *excess* and OUT of season.

Wherever you are in the world, specific foods will flourish and grow. Those are the *best* foods for your physical body. We believe we are supposed to be eating vegetables and fruits all day, every day, all year long. But, if you are living in a cold or temperate climate, I'm going to ask you to rethink that.

Vegetables and fruits, although they are healthful foods, are generally cooling in nature. If you are feeling cold (as most thyroid clients complain), consider eating fewer vegetables, and certainly fewer RAW vegetables, until your body rebalances itself and warms up. This could take two months, or two years, or longer depending on how much damage (imbalance) has been done.

Vegetables are categorized according to which part of the plant is generally eaten. Some vegetables fit into more than one category when various parts of the plant are edible. Some of the categories are leaves or leafy greens like bok choy, lettuce, watercress, cabbage, kale, collard greens, and parsley; flowers like cauliflower, broccoli, and squash; stems like asparagus and celery; bulbs that grow just below the surface of the ground like fennel, garlic, onions, and shallots; roots that grow into the ground like beets, carrots, daikon, and parsnips; tubers and rhizomes that grow underground on the root of a plant like potatoes, yams, Jerusalem artichokes, and ginger; fruits like cucumbers, eggplant, tomatoes, and squash that fall into the vegetable family; fungi that includes mushrooms like portobello, shitake, maitake, button, oyster, and truffles.

To know which vegetables are the best ones to eat at any given time of year, go to a local farmers market and see what's growing in your area. The produce will change all year round.

As I mentioned in the previous chapter, people suffering from thyroid disease need to be cautious of eating too many cruciferous vegetables (especially raw). This includes bok choy, broccoli, Brussels sprouts, cabbage, cauliflower, collards, mustard greens, and watercress. Sauté your broccoli and add butter and salt to get the best nutrition from it. And, roast those Brussels sprouts! They are far more delicious that way.

Keep in mind that you can eat raw vegetables. For example, eating a raw mesclun green salad with shaved raw carrots and beets would be great, but it may not be not wise to eat a raw broccoli salad or a raw kale salad. This doesn't mean you can NEVER eat raw kale or raw broccoli, it just means that you have to be a little more discerning with your food choices and understand how they can affect your condition, and then make the best choices.

Some other goitrogenic vegetables include cassava, daikon, maca, rutabaga, kohlrabi, and turnips. Cassava, otherwise known as manioc root, yucca, or tapioca starch, can contribute to goiter and thyroid disease unless it's been properly processed. Cassava contains prussic acid that can contribute to cyanide toxicity if eaten raw and in excess. Many non-gluten breads contain tapioca starch that is derived from cassava root. In small quantities your digestive system can handle that. In large quantities you may compromise your digestive terrain.

Daikon, rutabaga, and turnips are goitrogenic as well. Many years ago, when I first started my journey teaching people how to heal, I met a woman at a retreat. She had a HUGE goiter on the side of her neck. It was, hands down, the largest goiter I had ever seen!

When I spoke with her about raw goitrogenic foods she said, "Oh no! I eat raw turnips and raw kohlrabi all the time. I love them!"

I said, "Well, those foods don't love you. And, your body is talking."

She stopped eating raw turnips and kohlrabi and started incorporating sea vegetables into her diet. Two years later she was goiterless and gorgeous!

There are also some veggies I would like you to eat infrequently until your thyroid heals. These are nightshade vegetables and fruits (Solanaceae family) and include tomatoes, tomatillos, peppers, eggplant, and potatoes. Some people can have sensitivity to nightshades and may experience bloating, gas, diarrhea, painful joints, headaches, and depression.[99]

Nightshades, if eaten in excess, can inhibit calcium absorption. If you are suffering from hyperparathyroidism and your calcium levels are off, or you have achy joints and bones from arthritis, I would suggest eliminating nightshades for a while or reducing them to only one time per week until your condition improves. You can still enjoy tomatoes, potatoes, and peppers, just don't make it your everyday go-to food.

SEA VEGETABLES

Let's dive in and look at vegetables that grow in the ocean. The human body is made up mostly of water, both fresh water and salt water. To help us maintain a healthy internal liquid environment, we need to eat foods that come from the ocean. Energetically, sea vegetables are cooling and can help counteract "hot" conditions in the body such as inflammation, swelling, hot flashes, and high blood pressure.

Vegetables from the sea contain calcium, iron, phosphorous, potassium, sodium, zinc, magnesium, copper, chromium, and high levels of iodine, which is needed for thyroid health. Both too little iodine and too much iodine can lead to thyroid problems.

I've had many clients with hyperthyroidism, Graves' or Hashimoto's who think they need to stop eating iodine-rich foods, but

---

99   http://www.livestrong.com/article/367949-list-of-nightshade-vegetables-fruits/

it's not necessarily true. When I was first healing my thyroid condition, I had hyperthyroidism and goiter. Eating an iodine-rich diet was one of the steps that helped me heal.

Many clients who had goiters have reclaimed a normal-size neck by including sea vegetables in their diets on a regular basis, about one to two times per week. I do want to caution against using kelp tablets. I've seen lots of people actually develop goiter or Hashimoto's thyroiditis by using kelp and other seaweed tablets. It is too much concentrated iodine at one time, and is not balanced by other foods to make it easily absorbable. For example, a delicious bowl of miso soup contains a variety of foods that help make it more digestible: miso, scallions, fish broth (or water), sea vegetables, shitake mushrooms, tofu, and other vegetables. It's not just a big bowl of concentrated *iodine*.

Sea vegetables also contain alginic acid that can bind with toxins and radioactive waste in our bodies and allow their elimination. According to a 1964 McGill University study published by the Canadian Medical Association Journal, kelp can reduce the intestinal absorption of radioactive strontium-90 by up to 80 percent.[100]

A client came to see me for asthma, not thyroid disease. Julie had a dry hacking cough. We altered her diet and incorporated sea vegetables to help moisten and lubricate her lungs and intestines, so it would be easier for her to breathe.

Julie really enjoyed eating sea vegetables. She said, "I can't stop eating them! I am craving them all the time." I advised her to listen to her body and eat what she craved. Her body knew best what it needed. Within a few weeks, her lungs showed improvement, and she was using her inhaler much less often.

But, three months into her new eating regimen, she said, "Something terrible has happened! My thyroid got activated again."

I said, "Wow that's amazing!"

She said, "No, it's not! Five years ago I took radioactive iodine (RAI) because I had hyperthyroidism. My thyroid is supposed to be dead!"

I said, "You could be the poster child for how food can heal the body! The sea vegetables must have drawn the radioactive residue from your cells and the high amount of iodine may have started your thyroid functioning again. We should celebrate!"

100 http://www.livestrong.com/article/367949-list-of-nightshade-vegetables-fruits/

She said, "No! My doctor warned me that I need to retake the radioactive iodine, or I will have a heart attack."

I said, "Your thyroid gland wants to live after being radiated. That's pretty miraculous. Can you ask your doctor if you can hold off for a few months?"

Julie told me she was going to see her doctor again the following week and would discuss this with him.

The next time I saw her, she told me the doctor advised her that she would definitely die of a heart attack if she didn't take the RAI for the second time. So she did.

Many clients have confided in me that they feel guilty and are filled with remorse after taking RAI or having partial or full thyroidectomies. In the "Deeper Truth About Thyroid Health" chapter, I'll share how to continue your healing process without your thyroid gland. For now, just give yourself a big hug and a whole lotta love—you are alive, you are perfect exactly as you are (with or without a thyroid), and that's what matters most.

We are all on our own paths doing things we need to do for our own survival. Always do what YOU believe you need to do to take care of yourself, regardless of what I say, and regardless of what any doctor says.

I know sea vegetables may be foreign to some of you, but they can be a wise addition to your healing diet. The one thing I would caution against right now is sourcing sea vegetables from Japan and its surrounding areas. Since the nuclear disaster at Fukushima in 2011, there have been numerous reports of high levels of radiation leaking into the ocean.[101]

Even *decades* after the Chernobyl nuclear disaster in 1986, radiation levels were still high and people suffered from high rates of thyroid cancer, anemia, reproductive disorders, and weak bones.[102] [103]

Let's send our brothers and sisters in Japan and Chernobyl, and any other place that has suffered a radioactive disaster, a whole heap of healing love. But, let's source our sea vegetables from less contaminated waters for the time being. I've given a list of resources in the back of this book.

101   http://www.reuters.com/article/2013/10/10/japan-fukushima-radiation-idUSL1N0I003120131010
102   http://www.sciencedaily.com/releases/2004/09/040902085844.htm
103   http://epirev.oxfordjournals.org/content/19/2/187.full.pdf

ANIMAL PROTEINS

Naturally raised pastured animals provide food that is nutrient dense. This group can supply a large dose of nutrition in a small quantity of food, and can enhance your strength and vitality. Animal proteins contain a wide variety of essential vitamins and minerals. It's not just our little darlings, the vegetables, that contain all the good stuff.

Animal proteins contain vital nutrients that benefit the muscles, heart, and endocrine system. The thyroid combines iodine with tyrosine (amino acid) and converts it into T3 and T4.[104] A lack of protein is associated with hypothyroidism all over the world.

In my health-coaching practice, I've discovered that vegans and vegetarians often suffer from poor immunity, adrenal fatigue and thyroid disease. They rely on vegetable proteins, like beans, nuts, and seeds, which may not be absorbed as efficiently as animal proteins.

Energetically, most animal products and their fats from chicken, turkey, cow, goat, sheep, buffalo, eggs, and pork can strengthen and warm the body. Fish and dairy are the exceptions: fish strengthens and cools the body, and most dairy products cool the body as well.

Over the past fifty years, we have been taught that meat is carcinogenic, but that is simply not true. It's the quality of our meat and how it's prepared that determines whether or not it will contribute to poor health.

If meat is burned at high temperatures it forms heterocyclic amines (HCA) that can be cancer causing.[105] With that in mind, it's best NOT to eat meat that is too well done or burned to crisp. That doesn't mean you can never eat blackened, grilled, or barbecued meat again, it just means you should eat that type of meat less often so your body is not constantly dealing with an onslaught of carcinogens.

Although animal foods are dense with nutrients and energy, eating too much can congest the detoxification organs, and make your system sluggish. Again, an important aspect to remember when eating animal food, or any food actually, is "quantity changes quality." Many foods from both the animal and vegetable kingdoms can be delicious, nutritious, and health promoting, but if you eat them in excess they can do more harm than good.

104   http://www.endocrineweb.com/conditions/thyroid/how-your-thyroid-works
105   http://www.cancer.gov/cancertopics/factsheet/Risk/cooked-meats

For those of you who are having trouble digesting meat proteins, it's best to braise meats for long periods of time or cook them in stews to soften the proteins and make it easier for the body to absorb them. If you are feeling cold and can't warm up, red-blooded animals may be the best choice for you: lamb, beef, goat, duck, and wild game. If you are anemic, have low iron, are B12 deficient, or are low in vitamin D, organ meats like liver may be a good choice because they are rich in those nutrients. In the recipe section, I've included a delicious sautéed chicken liver recipe for you.

Eggs are rich in vitamins A and D, which are needed for endocrine function, but don't discard those yolks! That's where the vitamins are. Eat one or two whole eggs when you decide to have them, NOT a six egg white omelet and NOT egg substitutes.

If you are suffering from adrenal fatigue and digestive problems, bone stocks, rich in collagen and easily absorbable minerals, are liquid gold and increase vitality and energy. For many folks, supporting the adrenals with bone stocks naturally heals their thyroid conditions.

I worked with a client who was suffering from adrenal fatigue and goiter. She hadn't been diagnosed with hypothyroidism yet, but she was showing signs that it was coming. She began drinking bone stocks on a daily basis, and within two weeks, she felt better than she had in two years. Stocks are powerful nutrition!

I've worked with many clients who were eating fish as their main source of animal protein, and they were complaining of feeling cold. By altering their proteins and fats and adding more red-blooded animals and/or eggs to their diets, they began warming up. If you are cold, fish may not be the right protein for you unless you are eating whale meat. Whale is a warm-blooded ocean mammal so its protein and fat are warming rather than cooling.

Fish is great source of protein and is also rich in iodine; it can be a very good choice for healing the thyroid. But, you have to be careful with the type of fish you choose. Many fish, especially the larger predatory fish, like shark, tuna, swordfish, king mackerel, tilefish, and marlin, are high in mercury and polychlorinated biphenyls (PCBs). Choose fish that are lower on the food chain, anchovies, butterfish, flounder, hake, herring, mullet, perch, pollock, sardines, sole, shrimp, trout, crustaceans, and shellfish (lobster, crab, crayfish, shrimp, clams, oysters, scallops, mussels), as they generally contain lower levels of mercury and PCBs. Shellfish, by the way, are a good choice because they are also extremely high in zinc, which is essential for thyroid health.

When I was suffering from hyperthyroidism, I couldn't eat shellfish without breaking out in hives. Huge welts would pop out on my neck, face, and stomach soon after eating shellfish. Digestive problems, food sensitivities, and food allergies can be triggered by our inability to process specific proteins and nutrients.[106] My body couldn't process the high levels of iodine and zinc because my digestive system was out of balance. Today, I have no problem eating *any* ocean food. It's amazing what happens when the digestive system and the body get healthy.

Just as we need to source our land animals from great quality farms using traditional husbandry practices (grass-fed, pastured, naturally and humanely raised), we also need to source our fish and seafood from the cleanest water possible. I understand that much of our water is polluted, both the fresh water and the ocean water, and it's troubling. It seems as though we are making this planet as uninhabitable as humanly possible! Make the best choices as often as you can while you're here on the planet, and don't worry so much about everything. Focus on the things you *can* do to make your body and mind as healthy as possible.

DAIRY

I enjoy eating dairy products, and purchasing them from my local farmers. But when I was healing my thyroid, I took dairy out of my diet completely for two years! And, there is a reason for that.

Energetically, milk (from any mammal) promotes growth. It's designed to plump up the baby with as many nutrients as possible to help build their little growing bodies. I had a large goiter. The ideal diet for my thyroid condition was to take dairy out to reduce any more potential goiter *growth*. Whenever students or clients have growths of any kind (cancer, tumors, nodules) I advise them to eliminate most dairy from their diets for a period of time.

At the time of my diagnosis with thyroid disease and goiter, I was eating dairy ALL the time; it was a staple in my diet. I ate low-fat frozen yogurt almost every day. As a chronic dieter, I was mostly denying myself real food and real fat in my meals, so I was craving something comforting. Dairy is quite comforting. It takes you back to "mother" and

106 http://www.mayoclinic.org/diseases-conditions/food-allergy/basics/causes/con-20019293

to a sense of love and nurturing. Dairy is baby food and that's one of the reasons why so many people LOVE it. Many clients discover when they remove dairy from their diet, they lose that pudginess they've been struggling with or notice that their extra chin disappears.

You can witness the amazing growth factor properties contained within dairy proteins in body builders. They go crazy for whey protein in protein powders and protein shakes because it makes the body grow. If you don't want your body growing any more, ease up on the dairy, or eliminate it entirely, for a period of time.

I want to emphasize that I do NOT believe dairy is a BAD food. Dairy products have been used healthfully in many cultures and people around the world: Greek, Italian, Tibetan, Indian, Spanish, Swedish, Russian and many others, in the form of yogurt, kefir, butter, cream, and cheeses, from a variety of animals (goats, yaks, sheep, cows, water buffalo, etc.).

From experience with my own condition and those of many clients, I understand that if you want to inhibit the *growth* of any kind of nodule, lump, or goiter, take dairy protein out for a period of time. Once your body heals, you can add it back in, but in smaller quantities.

Dairy has many positive qualities, like making you feel plump. For those of you who feel withered or need to put on some weight, dairy could be ideal. One of the roles of mother's milk, for any mammal, is to populate the intestines with bacteria to help the baby digest food. Mother's milk also lubricates the inside of the body with a layer of mucous that helps us blink and breathe; not all mucus is bad. For those of you suffering from dry eyes, or a dry cough, high quality dairy may be a good option.

Excessive amounts of mucus, on the other hand, can cause quite a mess. Talk to the people suffering from allergies who are overwhelmed with mucus and blowing their noses every five seconds, and you'll understand what I mean. Their bodies are creating excess mucus because their food (whatever it is) is not being digested properly. The mucus acts as a protective layer.

I highly recommend cultured dairy products to help repopulate the intestinal flora and introduce a healthy layer of mucous back into the system after rounds of chemotherapy or rounds of antibiotics. Dairy is a great vehicle for carrying beneficial bacteria into the body and helping that bacteria *stick around.*

Naturally raised, grass-fed, organic, hormone-free and antibiotic-free dairy products can be good options for some people. For example, traditional cultures would cook oatmeal or porridge with cream or milk. According to Dr. John Douillard, both raw milk and heavy cream have NOT been homogenized. He says, "From the Ayurvedic perspective and that of many researchers, the homogenization process renders the fat in milk indigestible." The research indicates that homogenization, not dairy, causes lactose intolerance.[107]

If you're suffering from digestive distress, dairy products may *not* work for your system in their whole undigested form. You may need the milk proteins broken down, already pre-digested, in the form of yogurt or kefir.

I also do not recommend large quantities of cheese when healing the thyroid or any other condition. I know many of you are crying right now, "No! Don't take away my cheese!" Don't worry; it's just for a little while. Many people suffering from thyroid disease also have trouble with constipation, and cheeses, especially dry hard cheeses, can contribute to constipation.

As you can see, dairy products are not off limits once you understand how they can energetically affect the body. But, the only ones I would recommend at the beginning stages of healing are small amounts of kefir, yogurt, cream, and butter.

PICKLES AND CULTURED FOODS

People around the world eat some type of pickle or fermented food: in Japan, it's takuan pickles, oshinko pickles, and umeboshi plums; Koreans thrive on kimchi; the Europeans eat dill pickles, sour pickles, and garlic pickles; Germans are known for their sauerkraut; Russians eat kefir and pickled cabbage; and people throughout the Mediterranean dine on olives, pickled vegetables, and yogurt.

Humans fermented and pickled foods to preserve them, but other important chemical reactions took place as well. Fermented foods are probiotics that promote the growth of healthy bacteria. They also increase overall nutrition of food, aid digestion, and support the immune system. Probiotics are essential to good health. Probiotics are now

---

107 http://lifespa.com/stop-eating-dairy-until-you-read-this-report/

especially necessary to combat the widespread abuse of antibiotics, birth control pills, and other prescription medications that wipe out healthy intestinal flora.

Heating or cooking fermented foods can destroy beneficial bacteria and enzymes. Recolonizing the intestines with good bacteria begins with eating *raw*, unpasteurized fermented products. These are generally found in the refrigerated section of the health food store or market. For those of you who cannot tolerate cultured milk products (yogurt, kefir, buttermilk), fermented veggies are excellent for reinvigorating digestive health.

If you want to make your own sauerkraut or pickles, I've provided a recipe for you. But if you don't have the time or energy to make your own pickles, simply purchase them.

Sauerkraut and kimchi are both made with cabbage. The fermentation process does NOT entirely eliminate cabbage's goitrogenic properties. If you are eating these foods in small quantities (1 to 3 tablespoons per day) and you have a diet that is sufficient in iodine, your thyroid probably won't be negatively affected, and your digestive system can highly benefit.

I had a client with hypothyroidism who was suffering from constipation for many years. Her system was so sluggish that she could go to the bathroom only once every three or four days. Do you have any idea how toxic that could make your body? Lord have mercy! Unfortunately, many folks have trouble going to the bathroom, especially if they have been chronic dieters. This bathroom-challenged client started incorporating raw sauerkraut into her diet. At first she didn't enjoy the sour flavor. But, within two weeks, she started pooping on a daily basis, and by the end of the month she actually lost ten pounds! That's a LOT of pooping! Okay, let's get out of the toilet and get into the next category.

FRUIT

Fruit is succulent and sweet and energetically cooling and cleansing. Many people suffering from thyroid conditions often complain of feeling cold. If you're eating large amounts of fruit, pull back your intake to one piece per day or less, and remember to eat locally and seasonally.

I live in the northeastern United States where fruit does not grow during the cold winter months. Regardless of what the scientific studies tell me about the phytonutrients and antioxidants in fruit, I know that it is not the ideal food for me during the winter. This doesn't mean I don't eat fruit in the winter—I do. But, I eat it in small quantities, and I eat fruit that is indigenous to my environment. I do NOT regularly eat mangos and bananas in February in New York. Those are tropical fruits and contain way too much sugar for my system to handle, so I eat them only occasionally.

For the best-tasting fruit, remember to eat locally and seasonally. On a brisk fall day in the northeastern United States, a fresh, crisp apple will taste perfectly delicious because it's apple season. The apple is exactly what Earth is providing at that time of year in that environment. The apples are practically falling off the trees and hitting people on the head!

During the summer in southern Florida, it's mango season, and the fruit drops off the trees right into people's backyards. Wherever you are, eat the fruit that grows there, in the season it is available.

Peaches, pears, and strawberries consistently come up on goitrogenic food lists. You may want to reduce these fruits until your thyroid heals, but don't eliminate them entirely, especially if you enjoy them.

When I was growing up, I used to break out in swollen red hives all over my stomach whenever I ate strawberries. It was horrible! I LOVED strawberries. Today, I do not break out in hives from strawberries. Maybe it's due to the quality of strawberries, or maybe it's due to healing my digestive system? I don't know, I only know how my body is reacting today. Start paying attention to your own body and see how it reacts to food.

NUTS AND SEEDS

Nuts and seeds are great snacks and a rich source of nutrients. They are a better snack choice than pretzels, crackers, chips, or any of those "healthful" protein bars that contain unhealthful soy and other crap. But, just like grains and beans, nuts and seeds contain antinutrients in their skins that can wreak havoc on the digestive system.

Many years ago, I met a woman from India. We got to talking about health, and she asked me what I like to snack on. I pulled a bag of nuts and seeds out of my pocket and said, "I snack on nuts and seeds because they are healthy."

She looked into the bag and saw almonds with the skins on them and said, "You eat almonds with skins on?"

I said, "Of course! It's a whole food."

She said, "In my country, we soak almonds and peel the skin off. The skin irritates the digestive system."

I didn't understand the connection between almond skins and potential digestive distress until many years later. I was teaching a thyroid health class at the Open Center in NYC; there was an older woman sitting in the front row.

Toward the end of my presentation she raised her hand and said, "I do everything that you say. I eat eggs with the yolk, I cook my vegetables, I eat balanced meals, but I was diagnosed with Hashimoto's and I don't know why. The doctor wants to put me on medication."

I said, "What are you snacking on?"

She said, "Almonds. I snack only on almonds, two handfuls per day. Nothing else."

I said, "I think the almonds may be contributing to some digestive distress, and that may be what is bringing on your Hashimoto's condition."

She said," Absolutely NOT! In my country we grew up eating almonds." She was born in Europe in a Slavic-speaking country and migrated to the United States twenty years ago. She continued, "My entire family eats almonds, all my grandparents and parents, everyone eats almonds, and no one has this condition but me."

I said, "How did you eat those almonds when you were growing up in your country?"

She said, "We soaked them overnight, blanched them in hot water, and peeled the skins off."

I said, "Great! And, how are you eating almonds while you've been living here in America?"

She said, "Oh!" And, she laughed. "I'm not doing that at all."

Bitter almond skins contain small amounts of cyanide as well as other antinutrients that can block absorption of protein, vitamins, and minerals. In small quantities, that little bit of poison is not unhealthful; it can actually stimulate the immune system. But, in large quantities, it can irritate the digestive system and create a host of problems. In America, we're eating almonds in very large quantities: drinking almond milk, eating almond butter, using almond flour in baked goods, and snacking on almonds all day. It's not healthful, especially if those almonds are not properly prepared.

I eat almond butter, but I know those almonds probably haven't been blanched nor have the skins been removed. But the roasting and toasting of nuts and seeds help deactivate some of their antinutrients. I generally do not eat raw almond butter. If you are frequently consuming nuts and seeds that are not properly processed you could be setting yourself up for digestive distress and autoimmune thyroid diseases like Hashimoto's and Graves'.

Nuts and seeds, when properly processed, can be a great addition to a healthful diet. The concentrated protein, fat, and fiber in nuts and seeds can keep the body satisfied for a longer period of time than many other carbohydrate based snacks.

Energetically, nuts can grow trees. That's a tremendous amount of energy! It's best to eat nuts and seeds in small quantities, a handful or two. It can be quite easy to sit down with an entire bag of nuts and pop handful after handful into your mouth. If you notice a lot of burping or feel bloated and gassy after eating them, then you have eaten too many, and it is congesting your digestive system.

It also takes large quantities of nuts and seeds to make peanut butter, almond butter, sesame tahini, pumpkin butter, or any of the other nut and seed butters. It's probably best to not have more than two or three tablespoons at one time, depending on your activity levels.

Peanuts, pine nuts, and flax seeds pop up on the goitrogenic foods list. Many clients tell me they sprinkle ground flax meal onto their food. That may not the best idea when trying to heal the thyroid. I know we've been told to eat flax because it's good for us, but that's not necessarily true. It is estrogenic, so if you are estrogen sensitive or have any hormone-related conditions like breast cancer, ovarian cancer, endometriosis, or fibroids, flax could aggravate the condition.[108] You can still eat flax, just don't overdo it. And, some folks tell me they add peanut butter into their smoothies. That's not the worst thing to do, but it may not be the best way to support the health of the thyroid. I personally love peanut butter and jelly sandwiches. It's a classic! But, I

---

108   http://www.webmd.com/vitamins-supplements/ingredientmono-991-flaxseed. aspx?activeingredientid=991&activeingredientname=flaxseed

don't eat them daily. Remember, everything in moderation, unless, of course, you have a severe peanut allergy.

OILS & FATS

Eating a nonfat or low-fat diet, in the short-term, can help cleanse the body and clear a congested system, but if continued for too long, it can do more harm than good. "A deficiency of fat can create a sensation of inner cold; and body functions may slow down for lack of warmth, and the tissues grow brittle."[109] Lack of fat slows metabolism and other bodily functions. This is important to note for hypothyroidism and especially for weight loss.

All of your cells are coated in fat, specifically cholesterol. Many food experts, and doctors too, have made a complete reversal about their once negative thoughts on saturated fats and cholesterol.

We need saturated fat and cholesterol-rich foods for good health. And, fat carries flavor! It's one of the reasons people on low-fat and nonfat diets never seem to be satisfied and search for snacks all day long.

People are so afraid of fat—it's incredible! Especially women. Interestingly, women have higher rates of thyroid disease than men. They also have higher rates of osteoporosis, and that's partly due to a diet too low in fat.

It's better to cook with saturated fat instead of polyunsaturated fat and monounsaturated fats, especially if you are cooking on high temperatures. Saturated fats generally have a higher smoke point and don't oxidize as easily with heat.

For example, olive oil has a smoke point of about 375°F. If you take your healthful foods and coat them in olive oil, or some other vegetable oil, and roast them at 400°F or 425°F, you are actually creating an unhealthful dish. Rancid and oxidized oils contribute to inflammation.

My advice is NOT to be afraid of fat, especially when healing your thyroid. Fat-soluble vitamins A, D, E, K and B12 are imperative for proper functioning of the endocrine system.

Phyllis was a client who was deathly afraid of saturated fat, and didn't eat it for a very long time—25 years to be exact! She was also

109   Food and Healing, Annemarie Colbin, Random House 1986, pg 195

suffering from terrible bouts of depression and exhaustion. Reluctantly, on my recommendation, she added butter back into her diet.

After two weeks, she noticed she felt happier. She called me and said, "I don't know what the heck is going on, but I think *butter* makes me feel really happy."

Her body had been deficient in vitamins and minerals, and butter was the transporter for those nutrients into her system. Of course she felt better! When we get what we need on a deep supportive level, our bodies and minds run better.

Add some good-quality saturated fat into your diet while you are working on healing your thyroid: butter, duck fat, chicken fat, lard, suet, coconut oil, peanut oil, and avocado oil. Continue using monounsaturated and polyunsaturated fats like olive oil, sesame oil, and other nut and seed and vegetables oils, just don't overdo it. Steer clear of soybean oil, canola, and corn oil, or have those just infrequently.

SEASONINGS

This is where a lot of folks who take on a healthful diet and lifestyle go terribly wrong. They make their healthful food taste as bland and boring as possible. When that happens, eating becomes a chore rather than a pleasurable experience. Don't be afraid to spice up your food with herbs and seasonings. This will not only make your food taste delicious, but it can enhance digestibility as well. Herbs and spices contain essential oils that benefit digestion and absorption of food.

Many "hot" cooking spices were generally used in hot climates. Eating hot spices heats up the internal body, opening our pores to let us sweat, and cooling the body in the process. Hot spices work great in hot climates.

Many of the savory herb seasonings like oregano, basil, rosemary, thyme, and tarragon were traditionally used in temperate and cool climates. You can certainly mix and match herbs and spices to make food taste great. The recipes I will share with you use a little bit of all of these flavor enhancers to help make your food more digestible and taste totally awesome!

Healing your thyroid should not be about suffering through flavorless meals. It's imperative that your food tastes delicious, otherwise you're not going to want to eat it. I want you to fall in love with food and not be afraid of it or think of eating as a burden.

I had a client say to me, after she lost sixty pounds, "Who knew food could taste so good?" For years, Lori had been tormented by her eating experiences, and now she was loving food! It's a totally different experience to be able to enjoy your food.

Beyond herbs and spices, it's important to salt your food. Salt has gotten a bad rap, but salt is essential to all of your bodily processes. Humans have long revered the importance of salt. So much so in fact, that people were paid with it—hence the word "salary." Salt is as essential for our health as water.

Not all salt is beneficial to our health. Unfortunately, most of the packaged and refined food in our diet today contains high levels of poor quality salt. The refined commercial table salt that is in most food today has been stripped of its many essential elements and can contribute to high blood pressure, heart disease, hyperthyroidism, osteoporosis, and weight gain.

It's best to season food during the cooking process, and try not to salt your food at the table. When you cook with salt, it energetically has a different effect on the body. There are many different brands of sea salt to choose from. I prefer noniodized sea salt because I get my iodine from sea vegetables, fish, dairy, and eggs.

SWEETENERS

Glucose is fuel for the body and mind, but overindulging in the sweet stuff leads to serious trouble. A diet rich in fast food and junk food is dangerously high in refined sugars that compromise the immune system, adrenals, and pancreas.

Refined sugar can be defined as any "food" that has been stripped of its natural elements of vitamins, protein, fiber, minerals, and fat. To metabolize sugar effectively, the body depletes its own supply of vitamins and minerals.

If you are eating a modern diet that is filled with highly refined foods than you are probably eating a lot of sugar. Most processed foods disguise sugar on the ingredients list as dextrose, lactose, maltose, corn syrup, high fructose corn syrup, sorbitol, fructose, brown sugar, honey, sucrose, granulated cane juice, and malt syrup, to name a few.

One way to reduce sugar consumption is to eat more whole fresh foods instead of packaged foods. The further away a food is from its whole and natural state, the more sugar and other unhealthful ingredients it usually contains.

I am not suggesting you become overly rigid and eat a completely sugarless diet; small amounts of good quality traditional sugar can be fun. Stick with sweeteners that have stood the test of time, like honey, sugar cane, and maple syrup.

As far as desserts go, it's best to make them yourself, so you know exactly what's in them. If you're craving something sweet, you could always have a simple piece of fruit, even in the middle of winter, and even if it's not local or seasonal. Fruit can still be a good choice. It's nature's candy, for gosh sakes!

BEVERAGES

Drinking spring water, clean well water, or mineral water would be ideal. Those waters are loaded with minerals and trace elements that can benefit your health. Unfortunately, many of us do not have access to real spring water or unpolluted well water.

If I didn't know better, I would think we humans are creating a planet that only robots could live on, because they do not need to eat or drink anything to survive.

Many of us here in America are drinking tap water that contains both chlorine and fluoride. These substances are not good for thyroid health.

One of my clients, a dentist, warned me about the dangers of fluoride. She said, "Don't drink it in your water, and certainly do NOT put it on your teeth!"

Twenty years ago, I thought that was a radically wild statement, especially coming from a dentist. But, she was correct. Here's an interesting fact, "Fluoride does not accumulate in the brain. Of all tissues, the brain has the lowest fluoride concentration. It is generally agreed that the blood-brain barrier restricts the passage of fluoride into the central nervous system. The human pineal gland is *outside* the blood-brain barrier. It is one of a few unique regions in the brain (all midline structures bordering the third and fourth ventricles) where the blood-brain barrier is weak. Cells in these regions require direct and unimpeded contact with blood. Therefore, pinealocytes have free access to fluoride in the bloodstream. This access, coupled with the presence of hydroxyapatite (HA), suggests that the pineal gland may sequester fluoride from the bloodstream"[110]

Fluoride accumulation on the pineal gland has been linked to decreased melatonin production and abnormal pineal function, both of which alter the sleep/wake cycles and natural circadian rhythms. Bottom line: don't drink fluoridated water!

For those of you drinking distilled water, this may not be a good choice either as it is completely lacking minerals. When we drink water devoid of minerals, our body uses our own minerals to process it. Filtered water lacks minerals as well and may not the best choice either. I double filter my water to get all the crap, like fluoride and chlorine, out of it. To remedy this removal of beneficial minerals, I pour my double-filtered water into a gallon container, then add a pinch of sea salt plus liquid minerals back in to help it become more balanced. You can find a liquid mineral supplement that you can add into your water at most health food stores. Follow the directions on the container to figure out how much to add per gallon of water. This is certainly not ideal, but you have to make do with what you have within the circumstances we have created.

I do NOT suggest drinking spring water from plastic containers. As discussed, that water can be loaded with BPA that damages the endocrine system.

Other beneficial beverages besides water are herbal teas. If you are a regular tea drinker, like I am, you may want to consider buying tea in its whole form, instead of in tea bags. Many of those tea bags are bleached and contain chlorine. I know they are convenient, but if you drink a *lot* of tea, I would recommend getting a tea ball instead. You can pick one up at any kitchen supply store.

If you are suffering from adrenal fatigue or hyperthyroidism, caffeinated teas and coffee could make that condition worse. I've had many clients suffering from adrenal fatigue often complain, "But, it's only one cup of coffee per day! How could that possibly be affecting my body?" Newsflash! Coffee and other caffeinated beverages will make an exhausted condition worse. Even one little cup! You may feel an initial increase in energy, but you are actually drawing on deep energy reserves and exhausting your body further.

---

110   http://www.icnr.com/articles/fluoride-deposition.html

As far as alcohol goes, I'm not against it. If you are strong and feeling well, alcohol can be a fun addition to your diet. But if you are suffering from liver stress, exhaustion, fatigue, or blood sugar imbalances, alcohol can aggravate your condition. While you are healing, it's best to drink alcohol infrequently (only one to two times per week), if at all.

I'm a pretty healthy gal, and I have an alcohol-based drink one or two times per week. Around the holidays, maybe a little bit more. When I was first healing my condition, I didn't drink any alcohol. You have to decide where you are in your healing process and make wise choices.

Some people use alcohol to help de-stress. I've worked with both high-powered executives and full-time moms who are super stressed and who confide in me that they need alcohol to help them relax. It's not the best choice and may set them up for an addiction. Using alcohol as a substance to diminish stress and physical and emotional pain is a crutch. I encourage these folks to take a hot bath, and put a few drops of calming essential oils (lavender, orange, ylang ylang, frankincense, sage) into the water, or to relax with a cup of chamomile tea and a good book—even better, to treat themselves to a massage (my favorite way to de-stress!). Or simply to BREATHE, which most people do NOT do correctly. You will learn proper breathing techniques in the "A Deeper Truth About Thyroid Health" chapter.

As you begin applying all of this information to your life, remember to be patient. Changing the quality of your food can improve the quality of your blood, and that feeds your body what it needs in order to heal on a cellular level. Healing isn't going to happen after one magical cup of soup; it's going to take some time.

Now that you've learned a little bit about food, you can head over to the recipes section and start cooking. You may *not* be able to incorporate everything into your diet at once. Remember to always do the best you can and relax as often as possible.

To help you get through the challenging times, in the following chapter we're going to look at some botanical remedies that can help ease any discomfort you may be experiencing while you are going through the process of healing your thyroid.

CHAPTER 10
Helpful Herbs and Botanical Medicine

One of the reasons doctors prescribe pharmaceutical medications for thyroid disease is to help ease a patient's suffering. Unfortunately, many prescription medications can have negative side effects.

Medications for hypothyroidism and Hashimoto's can lead to rapid or irregular heartbeat, muscle weakness, irritability, tremors, impaired fertility, shortness of breath, nervousness, sleeplessness, hair loss, and decreased bone density.[111] Medications for hyperthyroidism and Graves' can cause skin rash, itching, abnormal hair loss, vomiting, swelling, joint and muscle pain, dizziness, drowsiness, decreased white blood cells, decreased platelets, and unusual bleeding.[112]

Besides a slew of negative side effects like the ones listed above, many synthetic prescription medications can contribute to liver dysfunction as well.[113] Impaired liver function can lead to higher estrogen levels and decreased conversion of thyroid hormone.

People may *initially* feel better on the medications, but within a few months or years, they often can feel worse. By taking the medications and *not* getting to the root cause of the thyroid condition, you may be jeopardizing your overall health and well-being.

Herbal medicine, on the other hand, is gentler on the body than synthetic pharmaceutical drugs. Many time-tested botanical remedies can help ease the suffering you may be experiencing, without a barrage of negative side effects, as well as support the body on a deep nutritive level. Herbal medicine has been around for thousands of years and is based on the use of plants and plant extracts that can be taken internally or used externally.[114]

There is amazing healing power in plants! Dr. James Still (1812–1885) advised, "I have long considered vegetable medicine all that is needed for the ills of the human family." That's my kind of doctor!

While my clients go through the process of healing their thyroid, I highly recommend herbal teas and other plant medicines for their additional support. Herbal remedies are subtle, so their benefits may

---

111 https://www.synthroid.com/whatissynthroid/sideeffects.aspx
112 http://www.nlm.nih.gov/medlineplus/druginfo/meds/a682464.html
113 http://www.ncbi.nlm.nih.gov/pubmed/10580751
114 http://www.drweil.com/drw/u/ART00469/Herbal-Botanical-Medicine-Dr-Weils-Wellness-Therapies.html

not be immediately noticed—which is part of the problem. We want everything to be fixed instantly, or at least overnight, after ingesting a food or herbal remedy. That kind of thinking shows a superficial understanding of healing that may not truly support the body on a deep level. One of the things I continue to emphasize, chapter after chapter, is our need for patience. Without it, we may not be able to heal *anything*.

Depending on your specific thyroid condition, these plant remedies can offer relief and healing:

Ashwagandha *(Withania somnifera)*—an adaptogen, which is a substance that strengthens the body and increases the body's ability to handle stress.[115] As you discovered in the chapter "Stress and the Adrenal Connection to Thyroid," it's imperative to de-stress, feel your grief, and support your adrenals as you go through the process of healing. Ayurvedic medicine, one of the world's oldest whole-body healing systems, developed thousands of years ago in India, used ashwagandha to treat age-related physical debility and impotence. It's also used for both chronic fatigue and anxiety. Ashwagandha acts on the reproductive and nervous system and has sedative and immune-strengthening properties.[116] If you are feeling stressed out or suffering from insomnia, reproductive issues, or exhaustion, ashwagandha may be a great herb to include in your healing regime. Ashwagandha is in the nightshade family of plants, so if you have a negative reaction or a sensitivity to nightshades, ashwagandha would NOT be the best herb for you.

Black Walnut Hull *(Juglans nigra)*—used to tone the intestines, and digestive system as a whole, and is especially useful for people suffering from bacterial overgrowth, leaky gut, and bloating. Black Walnut Hull is recognized as a powerful vermifuge and has been used successfully for expelling intestinal parasites and worms, as well as inhibiting candida overgrowth. Many people often complain of digestive woes and trouble with candida while they are dealing with thyroid issues. As you've already learned, when digestive health is compromised, it can contribute to, and exacerbate, a host of autoimmune conditions including Hashimoto's and Graves'. Candida is the friendly fungus that normally thrives in your large intestine (and can be found in trace amounts in other areas of the body). Trouble with candida begins when the ileocecal valve (the valve between the large intestine and small intestine) becomes

115   http://www.webmd.com/vitamins-supplements/ingredientmono-985-ginseng,%20 siberian.aspx?activeingredientid=985&activeingredientname=ginseng,%20siberian
116   21st Century Herbal, Michael Balick, PhD, Rodale 2014, pp 306-307

weakened by eating food that is out of season, abusing antibiotics, taking oral contraceptives that compromise digestive flora, a high carbohydrate and high sugar diet, and/or poor overall eating habits. When the digestive system becomes compromised due to weakened valves and imbalanced intestinal flora, candida can escape the large intestine to wreak havoc in other parts of the body. If you are suffering from a fungal overgrowth like candida, black walnut hull would be a great herb to get to know. It contains "sesquiterpenes" that act as fungal pheromones.[117] Herbalist Matthew Wood recommends one to twenty drops of black walnut hull tincture, three or four times per day. Start small, increasing drop by drop, until the intestines purge and then cut back.[118] If you're wondering what "purge" means, you may feel some intestinal cramping or experience diarrhea. Make sure you've got plenty of toilet paper on hand, and you'll be okay. While you're taking black walnut hull, or any other antimicrobial, antibacterial, or antifungal herbs, remember to be diligent about eating probiotic-rich foods, like kefir, yogurt, sauerkraut, and kimchi, to help rebuild and support the health of the intestines.

Bladderwrack *(Fucus vesiculosus)*—a sea plant administered as a tincture or capsule; it can be eaten as food or added to food, too. This plant is beneficial for both hyper and hypo thyroids, and is particularly effective for treating early-stage hypothyroidism. According to Dr. Ryan Drum, regular consumption of bladderwrack can also normalize a swollen prostate, lower chronic high blood pressure, promote healing and improve sleep. "Much of the iodine in bladderwrack presents as di-iodotyrosine, an immediate precursor of the thyroid hormones thyroxine and tri-iodothyronine. This makes it the sea vegetable of choice for treating thyroid disorders by providing the immediate precursors for T4 and T3."[119] I haven't had the pleasure of dining on bladderwrack yet, but I've eaten many other types of seaweed during my own healing process. I've shared some of those recipes with you in the recipe section. Ryan Drum suggests eating small pieces of bladderwrack with food, but for those of you who cannot bear the taste of seaweed, it can be ingested encapsulated in powdered form. Bladderwrack can also be taken as a tincture (mixed with alcohol and transformed into an extract).

Bugleweed *(Lycopus virginicus)*—an excellent remedy for hyperthyroidism and thyroid storms (soaring heart rate, blood pressure, and body temperature), plus hyperadrenalism. "Lycopus reduces the

---

117   Medical Herbalism, David Hoffman, Healing Arts Press, 2003, pg. 68
118   The Book of Herbal Wisdom, Matthew Wood, North Atlantic Books, 1997, pg 330
119   http://www.ryandrum.com/seaxpan1.html

output of thyroid-stimulating hormone (TSH) from the pituitary, turning down the setting on the thyroid level."[120] Many hyperthyroid clients often complain of an internal shaking that also makes their hands tremble uncontrollably; it won't stop no matter what they do. Bugleweed blocks conversion of thyroxin to T3 in the liver.[121] This reduces the amount of circulating thyroid hormone. If you are feeling hyper at night and cannot sleep, or are suffering from extreme nervousness, palpitations, heart-pounding thyroid storms, and/or internal shaking, put this herb to work on calming your system and your thyroid down.

Ginseng *(Panax ginseng, Panax quinquefolius)*—used in Traditional Chinese Medicine since 190 AD, ginseng is considered an age-old, time-tested adaptogen. Ginseng doesn't directly affect the thyroid gland, but it has been used to help boost immunity, increase energy and vitality, and alleviate chronic fatigue and adrenal exhaustion. Ginseng improves the body's resistance to environmental stressors and enhances physical and mental performance.[122] If you are feeling exhausted, this would be a good herb to take early in the day instead of drinking coffee, caffeinated tea, or other stimulants you may be using to help boost energy. Don't take ginseng at night or in the late afternoon, because it may rev you up. Also, keep in mind, this ginseng is NOT the same ginseng that you would find marketed and sold at gas stations, drug stores, and pit stops along the highway. That ginseng, in those little glass or plastic shot containers, is mostly sugar and caffeine. In the back of this book, I've provided a list of resources where you can find good quality herbal products.

Kelp/Kombu *(Laminaria)*—probably the most well known sea plant, and the first one I was introduced to during my healing process. Kelp is used as food in many cultures and also as a plaster (wrap) to reduce goiter. When I was healing my thyroid, Macrobiotic Practitioner Michio Kushi, advised me to soak two strips of kombu until soft, and lay them across my swollen goiter. Then I wrapped my kombu-coated neck with a cotton cloth to keep the strips of seaweed in place, and slept with it on all night. Michio suggested I do that a few times per week for a period of thirty days. Within that short duration of time, I experienced a significant reduction in goiter size. My goiter continued reducing even after I stopped wrapping my neck with seaweed. I was also eating kombu in my meals two to three times per week. Within eighteen months, my

120 The Earthwise Herbal, Matthew Wood, North Atlantic Books, 2009, p 232
121 Medical Herbalism, David Hoffman, Healing Arts Press, 2003, pg. 564
122 Medical Herbalism, David Hoffman, Healing Arts Press, 2003, pg. 545

thyroid had completely shrunk to normal size, and a goiter has never bulged out of my neck again. The kombu wrap that Michio Kushi recommended worked like a charm! Nature provides us with many materials we can use to improve our health; we've just got to start using them!

Lemon Balm *(Melissa officinalis)*—according to herbalist David Hoffman, "Freeze-dried aqueous extracts of lemon balm have been shown to inhibit many of the effects of thyroid-stimulating hormone (TSH) on the thyroid gland." That means it can be an effective treatment for Grave's and hyperthyroidism. Another traditional use of lemon balm is as an antiviral agent. Many students and clients suffering from thyroid disorders often complain of symptoms related to Epstein-Barr virus (human herpes virus 4), as well as frequent cold sores (herpes simplex). Lemon balm directly inhibits viral replication, and that aids the immune system and eases the toxic load on the liver as well. Melissa is a member of the mint family. It can be enjoyed as a calming cup of tea, as you sit back and listen to the Allman Brothers croon the classic rock and roll love song, "Sweet Melissa." Am I showing my age here? Speaking of ages, "In the Middle Ages, people used this herb to reduce stress and anxiety, promote restful sleep, lower fever, and ease the pain and discomfort of indigestion."[123] A simple tea would be 1 tablespoon dried lemon balm leaves, or ¼ cup fresh lemon balm leaves, steeped in 8 ounces of hot water for 10 to 12 minutes.

Motherwort *(Leonurus Cardiaca)*—primarily a "heart" herb, motherwort has been traditionally used for treating anxious mothers, promoting menstruation, relaxing muscle spasms, for uterine toning, and as a sedative for nervous afflictions.[124] This herb is excellent for menopausal women who are suffering from anxiety, as it helps drain heat from the upper part of the body. This herb is also used for people who have a highly stressed and freaked-out look, or bulging eye disease, from hyperthyroidism and Graves' disease. Motherwort is very bitter, so it may be best taken as a tincture for most folks. But, if you don't mind the bitter flavor, it is great as a cup of tea a couple of times a day. I enjoy drinking motherwort tea, especially if I find that my mind is racing and I don't feel relaxed. Use 2 teaspoons dried Motherwort per 1 cup boiling water, and steep 10 minutes. You could sweeten the tea with a little bit of honey to make it more palatable.

---

123 21st Century Herbal, Michael J. Balick, PhD, Rodale 2014, p. 204
124 http://www.susunweed.com/Article_Motherwort.htm

Reishi Mushroom *(Ganoderma lucidum)*—herbalist and cofounder of Arbor Vitae School of Traditional Herbalism, Richard Mandelbaum, recommends reishi for people suffering from autoimmune conditions like multiple sclerosis, lupus, and Hashimoto's thyroiditis. Reishi mushroom is an immunomodulator that both regulates and nourishes the immune system. It is also one of the best and oldest known adaptogens and was traditionally used to promote longevity and vitality. Reishi is revered in Traditional Chinese Medicine and is used to nourish the heart, calm the mind, and treat anxiety and insomnia. Many folks suffering from both thyroid disease and adrenal fatigue could highly benefit from using this adaptogenic immune-modulating mushroom. Reishi cannot be cooked as you would other mushrooms—it's hard and woody like the trees it grows on. It needs to be decocted (simmered to extract the flavor and nutrients) in hot water for a long period of time, about three hours. Like many other medicinal herbs, reishi has a bitter flavor. But, so does coffee and people drink that like crazy! If enjoying a cup of mushroom coffee sounds good to you, here is a recipe:

IMMUNE BOOSTING MUSHROOM COFFEE

- 16 cups (1 gallon) water
- 1 ounce dried reishi mushrooms
- 2 ounces dried maitake mushrooms
- 2–3 tablespoons ground chaga mushrooms
- 1/2 ounce dried astragalus root
- 1/2 ounce ground ginger (optional)

Bring all ingredients to a boil in a soup pot. Lower heat, cover, and simmer for three hours. Strain the liquid. Drink 1 to 2 cups daily for immune support. Mushroom coffee can be kept in the refrigerator for 5 to 6 days. Reheat in small batches (1 to 2 cups daily). Sweeten it if you need to.

There are many other botanical remedies that can aid in supporting thyroid health. According to herbalist and flower essence therapist, Claudia Keel, the vibrations of various flower essences resonate with the throat and are generally strengthening for the thyroid. Claudia emphasizes that many mental and emotional states can affect bodily functions, and this is where flower essences work best—on the vibrational state of the emotional body. You'll learn about that aspect of healing in the following chapter, "A Deeper Truth About Thyroid Health."

Claudia commonly uses the following essences with her clients who suffer from thyroid conditions:

Lapis Lazuli—opens the channels of communication in the throat chakra; amplifies the ability to hear information from physical and nonphysical sources; clears confusion between hearing and knowing. This is a gemstone that is made in the same way as a flower essence.[125]

Lobelia *(Lobelia siphilitica)*—supports courage to express and speak the truth regarding one's self; relieves shyness or shame around expressing one's self; controls misuse of energy; soothes throat-centered imbalances, and thyroid disorders.[126]

Golden Amaranthus *(Amaranthus hypochondriacus)*—supports learning to let go of overcontrol: "let go and let God"; tunes into the ease of life; develops ways to flow with the currents; eases transitions; strengthens the immune system.[127]

Motherwort *(Leonurus Cardiaca)*—encourages strength, assertiveness, and setting healthy boundaries; balances inner softness with strength; aids in knowing the power of one's feminine energies (both men and women); helps to soften hardened personalities.[128]

Essences are gentle subtle energy remedies from nature that do NOT interact with pharmaceuticals, herbs, or other remedies. Please keep in mind, however, that not ALL botanical remedies are good for all conditions, and some may be contraindicated.

A woman who had taken my Nourishing Thyroid Health Program sent me an email filled with extra exclamation marks!!! She said she stopped taking her hyperthyroidism medication and was feeling fantastic!!! But after one month, she began suffering from heart palpitations and anxiety!!! I inquired whether she was still following the recommended diet and lifestyle protocol from the program, and she assured me she was.

When I asked whether she was taking any additional herbs or supplements, she said, "My homeopath recently put me on an herb called blue flag."

125 http://alaskanessences.com/products/lapis-lazuli
126 http://www.deltagardens.com
127 http://www.deltagardens.com
128 http://www.deltagardens.com

After researching blue flag (*Iris versicolor*), I discovered it could be contraindicated in hyperthyroidism.[129] According to herbalist Matthew Wood, "In large doses Iris is a cathartic with toxic side effects. In small doses (one to ten drops), it flushes sugar from the liver."[130] I shared that information with my client, and she stopped taking the herb. Within twenty-four hours, her thyroid normalized again. The dose she was taking could have been too high, and/or her liver could have been flushing sugar, and that may have contributed to a hyper sensation in her body.

When using plant medicine of any kind, from the sea or from the land, it's best to work with a knowledgeable practitioner. If you live in the United States, you can locate an herbalist near you by visiting The American Herbalist Guild online (http://www.americanherbalistsguild.com). And, in the resources section of this book, I'll share with you some of my favorite practitioners.

If you begin reducing your prescription medications, please take it slowly. Work with a functional pharmacist or an integrative practitioner. Karyn Bender, the pharmacist in my online program, advises that you can get off your thyroid medications whenever you are ready. Keep in mind this is recommended *only* if you still have a thyroid. If you do not have a thyroid due to RAI or thyroidectomy, you would need to remain on some type of thyroid hormone replacement therapy.

When clients ask me if they should get off their meds, I recommend cutting their dosages in half, and then giving their bodies three months to catch up. Their internal systems need time to readjust the hormone levels, and that takes time. They may initially feel unbalanced: extra speedy if hyper or extra slow if hypo. But, that eventually normalizes because the body always seeks balance. After three months, they can cut the medication in half once again, and give themselves another three months to normalize. Soon enough, the physical body will begin doing what it is designed to do—function optimally.

After adopting the diet and lifestyle recommendations that I have been sharing with you in this book, many participants in my online program report back that their doctors have naturally had to lower their medications because their thyroid hormone levels began changing. I've heard the myth from patients and medical professionals alike that once

129   http://www.herbalextractsplus.com/blue-flag.html
130   The Book of Herbal Wisdom, Matthew Wood, North Atlantic Books 1997, pg. 320

you're on medication for thyroid disease, you can never get off of it. Many of my students and clients have already debunked that myth. The only people who need to remain on thyroid hormones for the rest of their lives are those who no longer have a thyroid due to RAI or thyroidectomy.

When people take any medications, including herbal remedies, the body has to process toxic residues. This can contribute to liver stress. It's one of the reasons liver enzymes are checked when you're taking medications for long periods of time. When the liver is not functioning optimally, the hormones can grow out of balance, and the body's natural detoxification system can become sluggish or weak.

As you are going through the process of healing the thyroid, it would be wise to do a gentle liver cleanse to support your body. But, if you are in a state of deficiency, as in the case of adrenal fatigue, hold off on cleansing until you rebuild and strengthen your system using the suggestions from Chapter 3, "Stress and The Adrenal Connection to Thyroid."

I highly recommend doing some type of liver cleansing at least one time per year, every year, as long as you are alive. This will not only assist your liver, but all other organs as well. It doesn't need to be anything dramatic, like a liver or gallbladder flush, where you purge your system, although I do recommend that for some people when it's appropriate.

A liver cleanse could be as simple as a juice fast for a period of three to five days, or fasting entirely, ingesting only water for forty-eight to seventy-two hours. I would recommend water fasting only if you have practiced this before. It's not for everyone. If you do a water fast, you may experience extreme headaches, pain, and nausea as your body begins purging toxins and waste.

Below is a simple recipe for a gentle Liver Cleanse:

LIVER CLEANSE

This recipe is for approximately one large serving of juice.

- 1 beet
- 6–7 carrots
- 2 inches fresh turmeric or ginger
- 1 green apple
- 1 cup parsley
- 1 lemon, peeled
- 1 tablespoon apple cider vinegar
- 1–2 pinches cayenne pepper
- ¼ teaspoon milk thistle tincture or extract
- ¼ teaspoon dandelion root tincture or extract

Juice the beet, carrots, turmeric, apple, parsley, and lemon in a juicer. Add the vinegar, cayenne pepper, milk thistle, and dandelion root.

Drink this juice three to four times per day for three to five days while abstaining from solid food. You could triple the recipe and keep it in the refrigerator, tightly sealed, and drink it throughout the day. It would be best to make a fresh batch each day of your cleanse. You could enjoy herbal teas (mint, chamomile, and lemon balm) as often as you would like throughout this cleanse. Milk thistle is an herb with a long history of being used for liver health, and it is now being researched as an herb for kidney health as well. The optimum functioning of the liver and kidneys is essential to helping your body naturally detoxify and heal. Dandelion has been used to help detoxify the liver, gallbladder, and kidneys.[131] It has powerful diuretic effects, which is something you want when you are intentionally cleansing. To keep your bowels moving during this process, incorporate yellow dock tincture: ¼–½ teaspoon 3 times per day. Yellow dock was traditionally used as a blood purifier and general detoxifier, especially for the liver.[132] It stimulates bile production and helps move lingering waste from the digestive tract. This simple juice and herb cleanse can help ease the load on the digestive system and

131 21st Century Herbal, Michael J. Balick, PhD, Rodale 2014, p. 280
132 http://www.globalhealingcenter.com/natural-health/benefits-of-yellow-dock-root/

support the health of both the liver and kidneys. If you are pregnant, I do NOT recommend any type of cleansing until after the baby is born and you have finished breast-feeding.

For those of you considering a much stronger cleanse, below is a recipe for a liver and gallbladder flush. This specific flush, I would recommend for someone who has a strong physical body because it can be draining and exhausting as your body forcefully relieves itself of congestion and possible stones. I would NOT advise doing the liver and gallbladder flush without doing a bug or parasite cleanse first, otherwise you may feel terribly sick. Once again, do not do this flush, or any type of cleansing, if you are pregnant, breast-feeding, or in a state of deficiency.

The recipe is adapted from Dr. Hulda Clark:

LIVER AND GALLBLADDER FLUSH

- ½ cup olive oil
- Juice of 1 pink grapefruit or 3 lemons
- L-Ornithine capsules
- Epsom Salts

Choose a day for your flush that you will be able to rest the following day. Eat a no-fat, no-animal-protein breakfast. Do NOT eat anything after 2:00 p.m. At 6:00 p.m., take 1 tablespoon Epsom salts with 6–8 ounces cold water. At 8:00 p.m., take 1 tablespoon of Epsom salts with 6–8 ounces cold water. At 10:00 p.m., combine the olive oil and citrus juice, and drink it all within ten minutes. Take four L-ornithine capsules with your olive oil drink. Go to the bathroom before going to bed. Get into bed and go to sleep shortly (within 20 minutes) after drinking the oil/juice mixture. When you wake the next morning, you will have to go to the bathroom. Expect soft stool and then diarrhea. Make sure you have plenty of toilet paper on hand, because you will probably be going to the bathroom many times throughout the day.

Both my husband and I, and countless clients and students, have tried this flush. It's dramatic and you may feel uncomfortable and nauseated the first day. But beyond that, it can help to provide relief to a congested liver and gallbladder and can help keep your liver and digestive system flowing more smoothly.

For anyone suffering with autoimmune thyroid conditions, I highly recommend a bug-killing and deworming protocol. Most folks have some type (or many types) of little creatures living inside their bodies. It's nothing to be grossed out about, it's just part of being alive. Animals and humans, and plants too, make great hosts for bacteria, worms, bugs, and parasites. Mostly, we don't even know they are there because the immune system keeps them in check. But, when their populations grow too large, they begin wreaking havoc inside the body. Some symptoms of parasite infection include diarrhea, constipation, bloating, excessive gas, cramping, bloody stool, anemia, swollen eyelids, itchy anus, skin rashes, and nausea.[133] To find a parasite or bug cleanse, go to your local health food market or herbal store, and inquire if they have an herbal "bug/parasite" cleanse formula. It may include wormwood, black walnut hull, clove, oregano oil, garlic, bayberry, quassia bark, among others. Follow the directions, and give yourself at least three weeks on the herbal protocol. While you are doing the bug-killing protocol, it's imperative that you recolonize your intestines with good bacteria (yogurt, kefir, sauerkraut, kimchi) and keep sugar to a minimum. Depending on which kind of little creatures are inhabiting your system, you may be able to see them on their way out. Mostly they are tiny and microscopic and will pass through unnoticed, but in the case of round worms and flukes, you may see them in the bowl before you flush. For general good health, it's wise to do a bug and deworming protocol at least once per year.

Beyond cleansing and flushing and buying stock in toilet paper, there is another level to healing that is absolutely essential and that has to be addressed otherwise your thyroid condition may keep returning at various times in your life. In the following chapter, we're going to dive deeper to discover the inner truth about thyroid health on the emotional and spiritual levels.

---

133 http://www.doctoroz.com/article/parasites-could-they-be-making-you-sick

CHAPTER 11
A Deeper Truth About Thyroid Health

According to modern medical science, our endocrine system is responsible for regulating growth, mood, blood sugar, metabolism, energy levels, reproduction, and immunity. The various glands communicate with each other through the production and release of hormones into the bloodstream. It's purely a mechanistic system.

But, there is another, much older, view that needs to be taken into consideration to truly heal the thyroid on a deeper level. According to ancient wisdom, those same glands and their positions within the body were referred to as chakras.

For those of you who are new to understanding the chakras, it is an energetic system within the body. You can't see chakras with an x-ray, and when they are out of balance, it won't show up on your blood test.

SEE 7 CHAKRAS ENERGY CENTERS ON PAGE 150

The chakras regulate and support your connection to your self and your emotional reactions to the world around you. There are seven main body chakras and each is connected to a different emotional, psychological, and spiritual aspect of your self.

For the purpose of this book, we're going to focus mainly on the fifth chakra and how it relates to the functioning of the thyroid, but I'll give you a brief overview of all of the chakras to help you understand your emotional body better.

The first chakra is your connection to Earth, your survival and ability to provide for yourself, and your feelings of safety and security. It represents your emotional connection to your immediate family: mother, father, sisters, brothers, grandparents, aunts, uncles, and cousins.

The second chakra is your connection to community and your significant others. This is where your ability to "feel" emotions lives, and it's where creativity is born. Humans can birth both babies and ideas from the second chakra.

The third chakra is your connection to your sense of self. This is related to your self-esteem and self worth: who you are and what you are doing in the world. It is your "take action" chakra! When we have a strong sense of self we can take on ourselves, and the whole world, too.

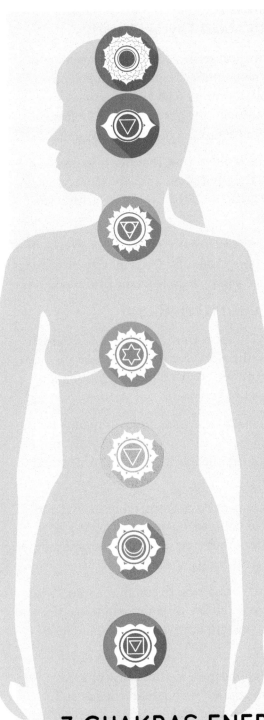

7th CROWN CHAKRA

6th THIRD EYE CHAKRA

5th THROAT CHAKRA

4th HEART CHAKRA

3rd SOLAR PLEXUS CHAKRA

2nd SACRAL CHAKRA

1st ROOT CHAKRA

7 CHAKRAS ENERGY CENTERS

The fourth chakra connects you to divinity or a belief in a higher power or god. It's also your connection to unconditional love, compassion, and forgiveness.

The fifth chakra is your ability to express yourself creatively and voice your truth. It's also connected to your senses of sight, taste, smell, and hearing.

The sixth chakra is your connection to wisdom and intuition. When the sixth chakra is healthy there is no second-guessing anything. You'll know exactly what you need to know. It's your ability to see and hear the truth.

The seventh chakra is your connection to spiritual nature. This is your present-moment awareness, your faith, and inner guidance. It's your ability to understand that everything is exactly the way it's supposed to be.

We are focusing our attention on the fifth chakra because it is directly associated with the thyroid, but please keep in mind that your entire chakra system (emotional/spiritual) can be affected by what is happening in any of the chakras. Contrary to the compartmentalized belief system we have been indoctrinated into with our modern medical model, all of the parts of your entire body are connected on many levels.

Physically, the fifth chakra is located in the neck/throat area. The color associated with it is bright blue. If you have an aversion, or a strong affinity for blue hues, it could indicate a need to connect more deeply to the fifth chakra.

There are some physical indicators that the fifth chakra may *not* be functioning optimally:

- chronic sore throat or laryngitis
- throat or esophageal cancer
- inability to make decisions
- repetitive throat clearing
- overtalking
- thyroid conditions or thyroid cancer
- lack of will power
- inability to express yourself
- swollen glands
- addictions

You can have an imbalanced fifth chakra, but not have any thyroid disease at all. It's just that thyroid disease happens to be one of the indicators that the fifth chakra is out of balance.

The fifth chakra is directly connected to our ability to communicate. A healthy fifth chakra is expressed through sharing emotions and thoughts that are truthful and honest. When the physical, emotional, and spiritual aspects of the body are in alignment, we speak with grace and wisdom rather than with blame, hurt, and resentment.

Generally speaking, if people cannot healthfully express their own personal truths, they can develop a hypothyroid condition or a goiter. The truth gets stuck in their throats, emotionally, and can create a corresponding physical condition.

In our modern worldview, many of us look to the physical condition first and treat that. This is one of the reasons why a condition may keep returning over and over again no matter what medication you use to treat it, or no matter how healthful your diet and lifestyle is. The root cause of the condition probably did not begin in the physical realm. Dense with matter, the physical world is the final place that a condition shows up. The thought or emotion that may have triggered that physical condition to start developing began in an environment that moves much faster, traveling at the speed of light, the world of ether and spirit. Let's take a look at some examples.

Diane, a student in one of my classes, was suffering from hypothyroidism and goiter. She told me that when she read and answered work emails she often found herself holding her throat.

When I asked if she was saying something in the emails that she didn't want to say, she said, "Yes! I work for a government organization, and I have to be politically correct with my responses." She realized that her standard email replies and the truth of what she wanted to express were in opposition. She was withholding her truth to save her job. She said, "If I write back what I really want them to know, I would get fired."

On the emotional and spiritual levels, if Diane hadn't expressed her truth, her thyroid may have always had problems no matter how well she was eating or how well she took care of herself. To fully heal her condition, she needed to actually get another job, one that was in alignment with her being able to speak her truth and nourish her spirit.

For people suffering from an autoimmune thyroid condition like Hashimoto's or Graves', it means their immune systems are attacking their own thyroid cells. The immune system is supposed to protect the body, not attack it! We need to look deeper to figure out why the protector would attack the body.

One of the reasons is simply that our physical cells are highly tuned in, via energetic and emotional vibrations, to what we say and how we feel. With any autoimmune condition, we need to hear where we are emotionally attacking either ourselves or other people.

Some of the things someone with Hashimoto's or hypothyroidism may voice either internally or externally:

"I'm not good enough."

"I can't do this."

"I can't believe I did that."

"I'll never be able to heal this condition."

"I'm hopeless."

"I'm a loser."

"I'm worthless."

"I didn't do enough."

"I need to do more so people will like me."

Oftentimes, we don't even realize the negative things we say to ourselves and about ourselves to others. It's an emotional and spiritual attack on the self. I would suggest you keep an "emotion" journal, and jot down what you hear yourself saying.

To heal this type of condition, it would be helpful to incorporate into your mind, heart, and body, the exact opposite emotional thought. If you hear "I am not good enough," that would need to be countered with "I am perfect exactly as I am." And, you will probably hear "I am not good enough" a thousand times per day every day. Every moment you become aware of that emotionally charged negative thought and feeling about yourself, it's imperative to counter with its opposite. In the beginning, they will just be words without meaning. But, after you repeat it enough, sending a positive message to your heart and mind over and over again, your energetic body will pick up on the new vibration and incorporate it into your cells. Even after years of actively doing emotional work on yourself (energy healing, talk therapy, etc.), you may *not* be able to disengage the negative thoughts, so it's crucial that they are balanced with just as many positive ones.

I often find that my clients who have Grave's and hyperthyroidism may be attacking other people, blaming them, condemning them, judging them, and creating a host of negative vibrations in the fifth chakra:

"He did this to me and ruined our relationship."

"You destroyed my life."

"It's because of her that I am like this,"

"My husband/wife makes me miserable."

"My parents didn't do what they were supposed to do for me."

"You are wrong, I am right."

"You are a loser."

"He is the reason I can't fulfill my life's dreams."

Blaming and judging others is deeply negative. Use your emotion journal to see how often you are blaming other people for what's happening in your life. When you hear yourself blaming someone for something, take another look and see where you can express yourself more healthfully. For example, if you say "He is an alcoholic who ruined my life," see where in that statement you can set a boundary and take responsibility for your participation in that experience. For example, "I do not allow alcoholic behavior in my relationship or into my life." When it comes to working with feelings and expressing yourself, always remember to keep it in the "I." It takes away blame and shame.

A student in my online thyroid program was suffering from Hashimoto's. She had read every scientific study about health, plus she was taking many classes on nutrition. She believed she knew best about natural foods and healing, and also thought she knew what everyone else in her life needed as well. She would constantly berate her husband and daughter, telling them that they didn't know how to eat well and care for themselves. The funny thing is both the husband and the daughter were fairly healthy. This student was convinced she knew the truth about food and healing, and yet she was the one suffering from thyroid disease, kidney stones, and gallstones. She was not healthy in her own emotional body and mind, and it was not only NOT working for her, but it wasn't working for the people around her.

Her arrogant way of being in the world was causing conflict in her relationships with her family and in her relationship to her own health. This is called spiritual sickness, and it doesn't get healed through food, not even the best food in the world.

Instead of taking another course in nutrition, she would have been wiser to take a course in acceptance, compassion, and understanding. Hashimoto's can sometimes manifest as, and stem from, an attack on the "self." Once she accepts and loves herself, it will become much easier for her to accept and love the other people in her life as well.

Be cautious with idle gossip and talking crap about other people. Healing disease requires HIGH vibrations; gossip is a very low vibration. It's one of the reasons gossip is mostly whispered in hushed tones. You may notice that people will either touch their throats or cover their mouths with their hands while they are gossiping. This goes for both the gossipers and the people listening to and receiving the gossip. Be discerning with what you say about other people, and the same goes for what you allow yourself to hear.

These deeper truths about the emotional and spiritual body can be accessed through using your intuition. Intuition is the "higher" voice inside of us. It's not connected to any religious belief, and it's not the one that blames and shames or self attacks. It's our higher consciousness, and for healing, we need to be able to hear it.

But, it can be hard to hear *anything* on the inside if we are constantly exposed to a barrage of advertisements, medical advice, product marketing, social media, politics, religious dogma, and mindless entertainment that influences us daily from the outside.

Through our senses, we take in all of the information that surrounds us. We see, hear, and feel everything we are exposed to, even when we are not conscious of it. Once we begin quieting the external noise, we can begin hearing that inner voice of higher consciousness.

One of the ways you can do this is by feeding your senses and mind what it needs. When the brain is properly nourished, clarity improves. My favorite way to feed the mind is with meditation.

Don't get nervous! Meditation is not scary or religious in any way. You don't have to sit cross-legged, wear a robe, chant, and light incense—unless, of course, you want to.

Meditation is simply learning how to focus your breath and quiet your mind. When the mind is quiet, you can hear what you need to hear, at exactly the right time when you need to hear it.

A Harvard Medical school scientific study on meditation says, "Meditation has been shown to affect emotional processing in the brain. These results are consistent with the hypothesis that meditation may result in enduring, beneficial changes in brain function, especially in the area of emotional processing."[134] Ancient people didn't have the scientific technology we have today, but they intuitively knew, without having to hook someone's brain up to a computer, that quieting the mind and connecting to the chakras through meditation supports the emotional body.

Meditation is not as hard as it may seem, but it does take practice and commitment. If you want to build physical muscles or have a body that is fit and in shape, you have to exercise or train at the gym. And, you can't just train one day per week, you have to train as often as possible for the best results. It's the same thing with meditation. The more you do it, the better the results.

To access this powerful form of healing, we start by simply learning how to breathe. The brain is the organ that requires the most oxygen to function properly, which means that breathing is brain food!

So let's start breathing. One simple breathing technique is to bring your breath all the way down into your belly, like a baby. If you watch babies sleeping, you'll notice they naturally fill up their bellies first when they breathe.

As we get older and life scares us, or we become afraid of things, we stop breathing down into our belly, and the breath lodges itself in our upper chest. If you watch a scary movie like *Jaws*, or a horror flick like *Nightmare on Elm Street*, you'll understand what I mean.

134 http://news.harvard.edu/gazette/story/2012/11/meditations-positive-residual-effects/

Fear causes us to take quick shallow breaths into the top portion of our chests... "Lions and tigers and bears, oh my!" I must've had lots of scary events (or events I perceived to be scary) in my life, because by the time I was thirty, ALL of my breath was up in my chest. I didn't take any belly breaths at all. Not one. I only realized this *after* I started practicing meditation. My poor oxygen-deprived brain was starving!

It was a real struggle to bring my breath out of my chest and down into my belly. I had to retrain myself every day for six months to release the bad breathing habit I created.

Try this simple exercise right now. Take a deep breath and notice where your breath goes. Is it filling up your chest? Is it sitting high up in your throat? Or is it relaxing down into your lower abdomen? Take another deep breath and get clear on where your breath is.

Now, place your hands onto your belly (lower abdomen), and focus on drawing your breath down into that area of your body. Apply a little pressure on your belly to see if the inhale can push your hands away from your body as you draw in your breath.

You may find that your breath naturally wants to stay up in your chest. It's just a habit and that's okay. Retraining your body to draw in breaths properly is going to take some time.

All life begins with the drawing in of breath. When a baby is born, we slap its butt to get that little cutie pie breathing its first breath of air outside of the water world of the womb.

Once breathing starts, that human being continues inhaling and exhaling for its entire life here on the planet. Until finally, it reaches the last exhale, on the way out of the body and out of this life. It's essential that we learn to breathe properly while we are here in the oxygen world, otherwise our days may pass us by filled with fear and stress and without clarity of mind.

It's never too late to start the process of breathing properly. Let's start right now by taking three simple belly breaths. Breathe in and feel the breath coming in through the nose and into the body, filling up the belly first, and then rising up through the solar plexus (the area just above the abdomen), and then into the chest. Breathe out, contracting your belly on the exhale, releasing all the air. Take another breath in through your nose, feel the belly filling, and then naturally expanding the breath up through the solar plexus and into the chest. Breathe out, exhaling fully, contracting the belly as the breath exits the body. Okay, one last breath! Fill up your belly, expanding into your solar plexus and then your chest. Breathe out, contracting your belly, and relax.

If you don't get this right at first, don't sweat it. I actually had to take breathing classes and practice every day for months. Be patient. I've said it in every chapter, and I'll say it again here. Patience is the key to understanding and healing the body on a deeper level.

Proper breathing helps fully oxygenate your whole body, which is great nutrition for all of your cells, especially your brain. Proper breathing also helps relax your nervous system and lower stress levels. There was a participant in my Nourishing Thyroid Health Program who told me she sat down and started focusing on breathing, and within five seconds she began to cry. Janice realized that she had been neglecting herself and putting everyone else's needs first. Simply stopping to breathe connected her to a deeper truth, and it was a painful realization.

Now, that you've taken three simple breaths, let me share what a quick and easy meditation could look like. You can practice this meditation exactly where you are right now. Whether you are sitting in a chair, on the couch, or even on the bus, anywhere works.

Keep your back straight up in the chair. No slouching. Sense your feet, and wiggle your toes around a bit. Let your feet and toes relax. Now, notice your butt sitting in the chair and feel your back against the chair. Relax your shoulders and rest your hands in your lap.

Read through this exercise first and then whenever you're ready, you're going to put down this book and close your eyes for a quickie meditation. Whether your breath ascends into your chest, or travels down into your belly, try not to worry too much about it. Worry will always stop you from relaxing into a meditation practice.

Sit in your chair and breathe ten simple breaths. That means ten full inhalations and ten full exhalations. I like to count down from ten to one. You can keep your eyes open or you can close them so you don't have any distractions.

As you breathe in, feel the cool air coming into your nostrils, traveling down the back of your throat and going deep into your lower abdomen. Breathe out and follow your breath traveling up from deep in your belly and out through your nostrils. You may feel cool air on your hands as you exhale.

While you're breathing, focus your attention on your sense of hearing. Notice the sounds you hear around you. Is there ambient noise in the background like doors opening and closing, traffic, birds tweeting, or dogs barking? Notice any sounds you hear coming from inside you. Do you hear a ringing? Is there a low buzzing sound?

Notice what you hear, but don't attach anything to it. They are all just sounds. While you focus on breathing, keep listening to the sounds around you. If any thoughts come up, notice what they are, but don't hold onto them. Let them come in and out, just like your breath. And, relax.

There's nothing to do except sit and breathe for a few moments. When you have reached ten breaths (either counting up or counting down), consciously feel your feet again. Wiggle your toes around. Feel your butt sitting in the chair. If your eyes were closed, slowly open them, and relax.

That's it. That's a simple form of meditation. If you could do that for five minutes every day, it could help lower stress levels, decrease the noise around you, and increase access to your internal voice, emotional needs, and innate wisdom. I often encourage clients to try meditation before deciding to take stress or anxiety medications. The benefits of meditation are far reaching. According to the *Journal of American Medical Association Internal Medicine,* mindful meditation eases anxiety, depression, stress, and pain.[135]

While you are relearning how to breathe properly and meditate, you may find that your mind becomes cluttered with erroneous thoughts. It takes training and practice to quiet all of that noise. If you choose to take on this type of practice, there are many great books about meditation you can read. One of my favorites is *Peace is Every Step* by Thich Nhat Hanh. He teaches that you do not have to "sit" to meditate; you could walk and meditate or do the dishes and meditate. The exercises are easy to incorporate into everyday life. It was the first book I read on meditation. It was given to me by my friend, Jason Poole, when I told him I was trying to find a way to "quiet my mind." That book was so simple and the practices so easy, I have since recommended it to thousands of people. There are many other great teachers like Sharon Salzberg, Pema

135 http://archinte.jamanetwork.com/article.aspx?articleid=1809754

Chodron, and Jack Kornfield. I love Jack's connection to the heart-based meditations. I cried for almost an entire year while incorporating Jack's meditations from *A Path With Heart* into my morning practice. Apparently, there were deep emotions I needed to connect with and painful memories that needed to be recognized and released from my system.

There are many great teachers who can help you train your mind. Give it a try and find someone you connect with who can guide you toward clarity and peace of mind.

The simple ten-breath meditation I shared with you was a first step to learning how to meditate anywhere and anytime, as long as you are NOT multi-tasking! If you are doing ten things at once, like many people do, you are cluttering your mind and making yourself very busy. Only when the mind is calm, can you gain access to deeper truths.

In earlier chapters, I emphasized how important it is for us to connect with our senses, especially when we are eating. Our senses of sight, taste, and smell are imperative to helping us strengthen and support the fifth chakra with the best foods for healing our conditions.

Part of the simple meditation I shared with you in this chapter, was focusing on your sense of hearing. People with hyperthyroidism and Graves' generally need to talk less and listen more. They have to become conscious of whether they are talking, talking, talking, and talking. It's time for them to focus more on hearing and listening.

For healing any thyroid condition, we need to sharpen all of our senses, especially our hearing and listening skills. Listening is one of the best ways to connect to intuition and our ability to hear the truth. When we hear the truth, it resonates with us on a deep level.

We need truth for healing. And, the truth is going to be different for everyone depending on where we are in our lives and what we're going through. The truth helps us figure out what is working for us and what is NOT working for us, and what to believe.

My client, Sharon, was suffering from extreme fatigue and hypothyroidism. When I first met her, she told me that she could barely get out of bed. We worked with her on her diet and lifestyle, and she began incorporating the recommendations I've given you in this book into her life.

Within two weeks, Sharon began feeling better and wanted to go for a blood test. I advised her to relax and be patient, because even though she may be feeling better, her blood work may show something completely different. Her impatience and "gotta-have-it-right-now" behavior pattern is one of the reasons she became exhausted in the first place.

Six weeks into her new diet and lifestyle, she couldn't take it any longer and went for a blood test. After Sharon got her test results back, she called me.

She said, "Oh my god! I just got my blood work back from my endocrinologist, and she said my thyroid is totally getting better. I'm sooooooo happy!" Sharon continued, "I knew it was getting better because I am feeling GREAT."

I said, "Fantastic! Now, just keep on doing what you're doing. You're on the right path."

Two months after that happy-go-lucky phone call, I received another call from Sharon. This time, she sounded completely deflated.

I said, "What on earth happened?"

She said, "I went for another blood test last week. And this time, my endocrinologist told me that I have to come into the office immediately, because my blood changed again, and this time it wasn't looking good."

I said, "I understand that. But, please tell me how your physical body is feeling today compared to how it felt three months ago?"

She said, "Well... that's the oddest thing. I thought my blood work would have been *perfect* because I've been feeling really, really, really good. I have more energy than I've had in two years! I have less brain fog and confusion, I get all my work done. I lost weight. Things were going so well. I can't believe this happened! This is awful!"

I said, "Please keep in mind as you go through the process of healing, your thyroid may swing back and forth like a pendulum before it becomes balanced and healthy. As you change the quality of your food and your lifestyle, your physical body is going to go through transformations as well. This is something most endocrinologists and doctors haven't been taught and don't understand."

Unfortunately, patience is NOT part of the modern medical protocol, and it's certainly not any part of our world today. Your blood may say one thing while your body is saying something completely different.

My own thyroid swung back and forth for two years. A happy healthy thyroid didn't happen overnight! Some of my clients have healed their thyroid conditions in three months and others in three years. People's bodies are unique and heal at their own pace. This is a deeper truth.

Check in with your physical body to see and hear what it is saying to you. Here are some questions to ask yourself every few months as you go through the process of healing:

- How do I feel today compared to how I felt three or four months ago?
- Am I sleeping better?
- Do I urinate less often during the night? Less often during the day?
- Any changes in energy levels?
- Do I feel physically stronger?
- What are my bowel movements like and how often do I have them?
- Is my throat/thyroid feeling less swollen and less uncomfortable?

As you move forward with healing your thyroid condition, you may also encounter setbacks with your health at any time. I'll give you a good example. Ten years after healing my thyroid condition, I was chosen for *Top Chef*. I started hanging around with the chefs and picked up some old habits that I had put down many years before. I began eating dessert with every dinner, and even having dessert with lunch. I was drinking caffeine again, about three to four cups of green tea per day, with big blobs of honey in each cup. I was drinking alcohol in excess. And, when I drink in excess, I crave cigarettes, and I smoke them! Within seven or eight months of incorporating those old behavior patterns back into my life, I crashed.

I went to the doctor for testing. She took my blood and told me the bad news.

She said, "You have thyroid disease (Hashimoto's) and you have to take medication. You may have healed this condition when you were twenty-eight years old, but now you're thirty-eight. Your body doesn't have the strength it did when it was younger. You're older now."

Her statement didn't resonate with me at all. Not one little cell in my body agreed with her prescription for my condition. I heard it with my ears, but my intuition said, "That's simply not true." I knew my current wild diet and lifestyle choices after *Top Chef* had directly contributed to my thyroid getting knocked out of balance.

The doctor's truth was that my body was too old to heal. My truth was that I needed to clean up my act!

So, I took action on the truth that resonated with me. I eliminated sugar and sweets, got to bed on time, stopped partying until the cows came home, and put down the cigarettes. Within thirty days, my thyroid tested completely normal.

My thyroid has taught me that it is a sensitive area in my body, and it may go out of balance again in my lifetime. I'm one of those people who have a compromised system from not being breast-fed, taking multiple rounds of antibiotics, and using both prescription and street drugs during my younger years. My sensitive thyroid is actually a blessing because it keeps me on my toes so I will take better care of myself.

We have to figure out how to access *your* truth and *your* internal wisdom so you can find the best path for your healing process, whether it's food, herbs, medication, surgery, or emotional and spiritual healing. You have the answers for you.

One of the ways to find the truth is to start questioning. French theologian and philosopher, Pierre Abelard, states, "Constant and frequent questioning is the first key to wisdom. For through doubting we are led to inquire, and by inquiry we perceive the truth."

An older student in one of my adrenal health cooking classes told me (and the entire class), that when he was growing up, you didn't question the recommendations given by the doctor. He said, "You just took their prescriptions, whatever they were, because the belief was, without a doubt, that the doctors knew best. They were trained by the best schools and had a formal education, so you didn't question what they said." He continued, "Today, I know better than that. There is too much money and profit involved in medicating patients. I question their motives for doling out so many drugs."

In my own practice, I've seen many clients whose annual physicals and blood tests were off, so they were prescribed thyroid medications. These clients took the medication without question, even though they felt zero symptoms of thyroid disease.

Some clients were scared, bullied actually, into taking medications or radioactive iodine even though they said they didn't want to take them. They overrode the messages from their own bodies and minds, because they thought the doctor knew best.

A twenty-four year old client came to see me for help with weight loss. Lori told me she was on Synthroid, but that she didn't actually have thyroid disease. Both her mother and her aunt had thyroid disease, so the doctor gave her a prescription for thyroid medication to help prevent her getting it. He also told her it would help with weight loss. Lori didn't lose ANY weight but she continued taking the medication because it was prescribed to her. She never questioned it and stayed on that medication for five years!

I've also had many clients who have either lowered their hypothyroidism medications or gotten off them entirely, and their TSH levels went up. That's normal. TSH is thyroid stimulating hormone. Taking prescription hormones for a hypothyroid condition makes your own thyroid lazy, or can put it to sleep. When you get off the medication, your endocrine system (pituitary gland) tells the thyroid, "Hey! Wake up little cutie! We've got some work to do around here. I'm sending thyroid stimulating hormone because I need you to start producing thyroid hormone. That's your job!"

Start questioning some of the medical protocols and always remember to check in with your own physical body to see how you are feeling. I believe that modern medicine has a great place in our lives. We have come a long way with our scientific and medical technology, but it is also limited in its perspective, and doesn't take the whole body (physical, emotional, and spiritual) into consideration. This is a blind spot in modern medicine.

Not only do I want you to start questioning the medical protocols, I also want you to question ALL of the things I say as well. I want you to question any other expert that is living outside of your body telling you what to do.

The truth is, YOU are living inside your body. Not me. Not the doctor. Not the expert. Your body will talk to you. When you are in tune with your body and you have learned how to quiet the noise through simple meditation and breathing, you can actually hear what your body is saying. This doesn't mean you shouldn't take the doctor's advice or my advice, it just means to listen to it and discern whether it could be the right choice for you. Don't get bullied into anything.

When I'm teaching or sharing information about food, lifestyle, and consciousness, I always tell my students and clients that they should try any internal "Aha! That makes sense to me!"

It's time to figure out what the truth is for you. Is it something you've read or have been fed by the experts or the books or by the latest scientific nutritional discovery? Or is it something that truly resonated within you?

I'll give you a great example. I went to a popular raw foods institute in Florida. When I arrived, the director of the institute performed a blood analysis to test my blood and see how healthy it was.

The woman pricked my finger and tested my blood. She looked at me and said, "Oh your blood looks great. How long have you been raw?"

I said, "Well I'm not really *raw*. I eat raw salads and raw veggies, but I also eat cooked food and fermented foods and animal fats and animal proteins. I eat just about everything except junk food and fast food."

She raised an eyebrow and replied, "According to nutritional science, raw plant foods are the ideal diet for humans. They are rich in enzymes and nutrients. When you cook food, it denatures it and contributes to cancer and other illnesses."

She gave me a long list of nutrition books to read to learn about the various studies on raw foods. Then she pulled out a piece of paper, and said, "And, if you're going to take on a raw foods diet, you'll need to incorporate these digestive enzymes, probitoics, vitamin B 12 supplement...."

On the paper, she checked off ten to twelve supplements for me to take to maintain a healthy raw foods diet. Just like when I was at the doctor's office and felt a wall, an energy block, come up between the doctor and me, it came up again with the raw foods lady.

Immediately, I questioned, "If a raw plant foods diet is the ideal diet for human beings, why on earth would I need all these supplements?"

She told me it was to keep me healthy as I transitioned from cooked foods to raw foods. It didn't sound reasonable to me. I stayed for eight days at the institute and tried the completely raw foods diet to see how it felt in my physical body.

By day four, I came to the conclusion that I certainly do LOVE a raw salad and fresh raw veggies, but I do NOT love them three times per day, every day, including snacks, PLUS shots of wheat grass. Truthfully, that amount of raw plant food made me feel quite nauseated.

Now, don't get me wrong, raw foods work great for some people and for some conditions, but not for all people or for all conditions. I encourage you to experiment with everything I've shared with you inside *your* own physical body to see how it feels. Experience is a great teacher.

We all have access to inner wisdom and truth, and we need to work it like a muscle to strengthen it. One way we can find it is through connecting with our intuition.

The definition of intuition is "a natural ability that makes it possible to know something without any proof or evidence."[136] That means you will know something without having to call to mind the *reason* you believe it. This is truth that goes beyond any study you've read, or the latest news story about the greatest supplement on earth, or the newest "superfood" on the market. Intuition is your internal knowing, and it's the deepest wisdom you have access to.

With practice, you'll know which healing modality to try for your condition: raw foods, cooked foods, massage, acupuncture, herbs, energy healing, psychic healing, shamanism, indigenous healing plants, modern medicine, or pharmaceutical drugs.

It's time to access your truth and inner wisdom. Remember the breathing exercise and easy meditation? We're going to do that again, but with a slightly different focus this time.

All the hyperthyroid folks and people suffering from Graves' disease are groaning right now, "Oh my god!!! If she makes me take one more breath and try to relax, I'm going to smash this book on top of her head!"

---

136 http://www.merriam-webster.com/dictionary/intuition

This time when you do the ten-breath meditation, focus your attention, with eyes closed, on the third eye or the pineal gland (sixth chakra). That's the area in the center of your forehead, just above your eyebrows. It's your GPS.

Relax your body to release tension, but keep your spine straight in your chair. Feel your feet in your shoes, and wiggle your toes around a bit. Begin the breathing process, and draw your attention to the area between your eyebrows. Breathe in and breathe out, bringing your breath all the way down into your belly, but keeping your focus on your third eye. At first it may feel like you are crossing your eyes, but you're not. You're just focusing consciousness onto a specific area in your emotional/spiritual body. Don't worry so much about where your breath is going this time, just focus on the area between your eyebrows.

I want you to put this book down, wherever you are, and take ten deep breaths focusing on your pineal gland. Right now, not at the end of the chapter!

How was that? Many of you may not have felt anything – that's okay. As you continually bring your attention to your pineal gland, with practice and patience, you will begin gaining more clarity, insight, and wisdom.

Meditation is like a muscle and the more you work it, the stronger it gets. We want and need the pineal gland to grow stronger and more active because it can help us better connect to our emotional, physical and spiritual selves. Inner wisdom can guide us, especially if we get stuck with our healing processes.

Many times I've seen clients get stuck on something they learned years prior; they can't let go of it. They get attached to an idea, whether it's a type of food or a supplement or medicine, regardless of how their physical bodies may be feeling. A healthy fifth chakra, supported by internal wisdom (sixth chakra), allows us to let go of attachment.

When I was studying macrobiotics many years ago, there was a woman in the class who was on a strict healing diet. She ate limited amounts of oils, lots of grains, beans, and vegetables, and fish only one time per month. It was a cleansing diet and healing protocol. In the beginning, it worked great for her.

Over the years, I would see her at various macrobiotic potluck parties, and she looked like she was growing frailer each time. Almost two decades later, she looked like a stick figure, just skin and bones, hunched over, suffering from bone loss, and covered with liver spots all over her skin. She was still on that same restrictive healing diet from twenty years prior, and it was having the opposite effect on her body. That healing diet worked in the beginning of her journey because she needed cleansing. But as her physical body changed, and then changed again, she never connected to her own internal wisdom to see what her body needed next to thrive. She remained stuck in that one frame of mind for many years.

That's where intuition comes in handy. It's the ability to SEE. There's a reason ancient people called it the third eye. The pineal gland or third eye gives you the ability to SEE the truth, and the fifth chakra or throat chakra allows you to EXPRESS that truth.

I have one final meditation to help you connect to the fifth chakra and energize your whole body in a healthful way. I promise it won't kill you, and it just may make you feel better!

For those of you who no longer have a thyroid, this one is especially important for you. Just because the thyroid is no longer there, that does NOT mean the energetic body, emotional body, and spiritual body are not functioning. If someone loses a body part or organ, the physical body may be altered, but the emotional and spiritual bodies still need support. We've all heard stories of people who lose an arm or a leg in an accident or a war, and swear they can still feel the missing part. It's often referred to as a ghost limb. It's the same thing with the missing thyroid.

We are much more than just our physical bodies. If we focus solely on the physical body, we cut ourselves off from the emotional and spiritual parts of our existence. This narrow focus, I believe, is one of the biggest contributors to recurring illnesses. So, whether you have your thyroid or you do NOT have your thyroid, the next meditation is a great practice.

After you start breathing, with your eyes closed, you are going to visualize a blue healing color or anything that represents health and vitality to you: blue water, blue crystal, blue sky, blue flowers, etc. It could be any shade of blue, and if another color pops up for you, that's okay. Breathe and visualize that color. I chose blue because, according to ancient healing and energetic medicine, that is the color associated with the fifth chakra.

With your eyes closed, send a smile to your throat area. Send it love. This is your area for expression, and it is here to support you on your journey through this lifetime. Send the throat love and visualization for at least ten breaths, and then open your eyes.

How was that for you? Did anything come up visually or emotionally while your eyes were closed?

Karyn was a client suffering from hyperthyroidism and Graves'. When she closed her eyes and visualized her throat area, she saw a red sports car! It was appropriate because a sports car is designed to drive really fast, and her thyroid was hyper (fast) and inflamed (red). For her next visualization, I suggested that she slow the car down a bit and visualize something that doesn't move 120 miles per hour, like a bicycle, a skateboard, a kayak, or a family sedan.

Another client, when visualizing her throat area, saw an axe, which was appropriate. Half of her thyroid had been surgically removed; she told me she felt like she had been chopped into. The axe represented how she was emotionally feeling. Her challenge was to visualize her thyroid as happy, healthy, and whole, even though only half of it was there.

I've had many clients tell me that when they do this visualization exercise and send love to their bodies and to their throats (thyroids), they cry. It's not often that we consciously send love to ourselves and to the essences and voices of who we are.

Many folks who have had their thyroids removed visualize the blue color and have told me that it's very comforting for them. The emotional body and the spiritual body are still whole and complete and need our love and attention too.

For the purpose of the this book, we've done only ten breaths with each short meditation. Ideally, it would be great if you could do the meditations for a longer period of time (fifteen minutes or more). Start with ten breaths, and as you get more comfortable, increase your meditation time.

As you can see (with your third eye!), there are many levels to healing the body. When I say body, I'm talking about the physical, emotional, energetic, and spiritual body.

As a whole, here are some of the various ways we can emotionally and spiritually heal our thyroids:

- Voice your truth, and remember to keep it in the "I"
- Express yourself in a healthy manner (talk positively not negatively)
- Consciously focus on your breath
- Get in touch with your intuition and inner wisdom
- Become aware of the senses on your face (sight, sound, smell, and taste) and how they relate to your food and to the world around you
- Trust yourself
- Send your thyroid a large dose of love

Throughout this book, I've shared with you a wide variety of information that can help heal your condition on some level: physical, emotional, energetic, and spiritual. Experiment on yourself.

I am proud of you for carving out the time to read this book and to take this journey for your health. I am sending you and your fifth chakra, and the rest of your beautiful body, a whole lot of healing love.

Now, get ready to set the table. It's time to feed your body delicious food that will give you the energy needed to support your thyroid and your body as a whole. I saved the recipes for the last chapter so you could work up a healthy appetite!

CHAPTER 12
Recipes! Recipes! Recipes!

Every day, I receive emails from people asking, "Can you tell me what to eat for my thyroid condition?" As you may have gathered from the information in this book, it's not that simple.

To figure out what to eat for any thyroid condition, you've got to take climate and season into consideration, as well as the way traditional foods were prepared and eaten in your part of the world. Proper food choices can fuel your body, benefit your pineal gland and endocrine system, and help you acclimate to your environment so that you'll feel more balanced and grounded.

I've got plenty of easy recipes, but you are going to have to do some research and make simple adjustments to make them the most nutritious for you. Recipes are only guidelines. You can adjust the ingredients in any recipe to make it nourishing for your body by using, as often as possible, the local and seasonal produce.

Answer these five simple questions to help you get reconnected to your environment and the best food for your body:

1. Where are you?
2. Which climate do you live in: temperate, tropical, subtropical, desert, dry, Mediterranean, cold, polar?
3. What type of produce grows in your region?
4. Which animal fats and proteins are, and were, indigenous to your area?
5. What traditional foods were eaten in your region of the world, and how were they prepared?

Once you understand your background, you can make any recipe healthful and delicious. You can certainly use the recipes exactly as they are, but remember to make seasonal and local food adjustments for the best results. Discovering how to use food as medicine can help you start feeling better in no time!

There is a wide variety of recipes: stock, beans, grains, vegetables, sea vegetables, animal proteins, and desserts. Pick and choose the recipes that call to you first—meaning . . . you may hear an internal "yum"! Remember to be adventurous as well; try eating some of the traditional foods that may be foreign to you.

As you go through the process of trying any new food, it would be wise to keep a food journal and write down how each of these foods makes you feel, both physically and emotionally. Remember to try everything at least once, and to experiment with what you eat. It's your body—have some fun and play with it.

The recipes I'm providing have worked for many people, but they may not work for you. It's time for you to begin recognizing which foods make you feel nourished and which do NOT, no matter how healthful the foods may seem.

You are living inside your body, and you are building your cells with every morsel of food you put inside your mouth. Get connected to your food and your body on a deeper level to begin understanding how the food you are eating makes you feel.

Get ready to get nourished!

BONE STOCKS

The first batch of recipes I'm providing is bone stocks. I recommend drinking bone stock to help support the adrenals, improve energy, and heal the digestive system.

According to scientific studies, the skeleton is part of the endocrine system and controls energy, blood sugar, and weight.[137] Many people suffering from thyroid disease can also experience bone problems like osteoporosis, osteopenia, rheumatoid arthritis, and osteoarthritis. Bone stocks contain easily absorbable liquid minerals, amino acids, and collagen, and can be highly therapeutic in nourishing your bones and endocrine system. Use stocks as the base for your soups and stews, or you could simply sip on some seasoned stock throughout your day.

There was a student in my Nourishing Thyroid Program who started drinking two cups of bone stock daily. Her energy levels increased dramatically, and her eyebrows began growing back. Many people suffering from thyroid conditions lose the outer third of their eyebrows. She was over fifty and never expected that her eyebrows would return.

After eight months of drinking stock two times per day every day, she told me that she couldn't stomach it anymore. She said, "I can't even look at another cup of stock!"

I said, "Great! That means you're full!"

There is going to come a time when your body will reject the same food that nourished you. Always listen to your body and let it guide you. That student will start craving stocks again when her body is ready, especially in the fall and winter when the temperature dips, and it gets cold. That is the traditional time of year when bone stocks were most often used. Stocks can be eaten in the warmth of spring and summer too, but those would generally be lighter stocks, like fish and vegetable. You can always eat some type of stock year-round to give your body a burst of deep nutrition.

---

137 http://www.medicalnewstoday.com/articles/79522.php

Iodine-Rich Fish Stock

Ingredients

Carcass of one or two white-meat fish (cod, scrod), about 1 to 2 pounds
4-5 quarts water
1 tablespoon grass-fed butter (optional)
1 cup white wine
2 onions, peeled and quartered
3 carrots, rinsed and chopped
2 stalks celery, rinsed and chopped
6 to 8 sprigs fresh thyme leaves or 2 teaspoons dried
1 tablespoon whole peppercorns
2 dried bay leaves
¼ bunch fresh parsley with stems

Preparation

1. Place bones and 4-5 quarts water in an 8-quart stockpot; bring to a boil.

2. Skim off and discard any foam or scum that rises to the top.

3. Add butter, wine, onions, carrots, celery, thyme, peppercorns, and bay leaves.

4. Reduce heat to low. Cover, and simmer 4 to 12 hours.
   The longer you cook stock, the more concentrated it becomes.

5. Add parsley during the last hour of cooking.

6. Strain the stock into containers; discard bones and vegetables.

7. Place stock in the refrigerator, and let fat congeal overnight.

8. Skim and discard fat.

9. Pour defatted stock into freezer-safe containers, but do NOT fill to the top—stock expands as it freezes. Leave at least one inch of space.

Basic Chicken Stock

Ingredients

Bones 1 to 2 pastured chickens (carcass, neck, wingtips, thighs, drums, feet, etc.), about 1 to 2 pounds

4-5 quarts water

1 tablespoon whole peppercorns

2 onions, peeled and quartered

3 carrots, rinsed and chopped

2–3 stalks celery, rinsed and chopped

5 to 6 sprigs fresh thyme leaves or 2 teaspoons dried

¼ bunch fresh parsley with stems

*If you want to make a turkey stock, swap out the chicken bones for turkey bones.

Preparation

1. Place bones and 4-5 quarts water in an 8-quart stockpot; bring to a boil.

2. Skim off and discard any foam or scum that rises to the top of the pot.

3. Add peppercorns, onions, carrots, celery, and thyme.

4. Reduce heat to low. Cover, and simmer 6-12 hours or longer. The longer you cook stock, the more concentrated it becomes. Add parsley toward the end of cooking.

5. Strain the stock into containers; discard bones and vegetables.

6. Place stock in the refrigerator, and let fat congeal overnight.

7. Skim and discard fat.

8. Pour defatted stock into freezer–safe containers, but do NOT fill to the top—stock expands as it freezes. Leave at least one inch of space.

9. You can freeze stock for 3-4 months.

Duck Stock

Ingredients

Bones of 1 to 2 free–range, pastured ducks (carcass, neck, wingtips, thighs, drums, etc.), about 1 to 2 pounds
4-5 quarts water
1 cup red wine
2 onions, peeled and quartered
3 carrots, rinsed and chopped
2 cloves garlic, peeled
6 to 8 sprigs fresh thyme leaves or 2 teaspoons dried
1 tablespoon whole peppercorns
1 bay leaf
¼ bunch fresh parsley with stems

Preparation

1. Place bones and 4-5 quarts water in an 8-quart stockpot; bring to a boil.

2. Skim off and discard any foam or scum that rises to the top.

3. Add wine, onions, carrots, garlic, thyme, peppercorns, and bay leaf.

4. Return to a boil.

5. Reduce heat to low. Cover, and simmer 6-12 hours or even longer. The longer you cook stock, the more concentrated it becomes. Add parsley at the end of cooking.

6. Strain the stock into containers; discard bones and vegetables.

7. Place stock in the refrigerator and let fat congeal overnight.

8. Skim off fat; discard the fat or use it for cooking. If you are going to use the fat, dry it on paper towels, and store it in the refrigerator. Duck fat is one of my favorite fats!

9. Pour defatted stock into freezer-safe containers, but do not fill to the top as stock expands as it freezes. Leave at least one inch of space.

10. You can freeze stock for 3-4 months.

Vegetable Stock

Ingredients

1 tablespoon olive or coconut oil
2 large onions, peeled and quartered
3 carrots, rinsed and chopped
2 stalks celery plus leaves, rinsed and chopped
1 leek, white and light green parts, cleaned and sliced
2–3 cloves garlic, peeled
1 teaspoon sea salt
½ bunch fresh parsley with stems
4-5 quarts water
5 to 6 sprigs fresh thyme sprigs or 2 teaspoons dried leaves
2 bay leaves

Preparation

1. Heat oil in an 8-quart stockpot over medium-high heat.

2. Add onions, carrots, celery, leeks, garlic, and salt.

3. Cook vegetables until lightly browned.

4. Add parsley, thyme, bay leaves, and 4-5 quarts water; bring to a boil.

5. Reduce heat to low. Cover, and simmer for 1 or 2 hours.

6. Strain the stock; discard vegetables, and store in airtight containers in the freezer.

If freezing stock, leave 1 to 2 inches of empty space inside the container for expansion as the stock expands as it freezes.

Beef Stock

Ingredients

2-4 pounds beef bones (knuckles, shanks, oxtail, or neck)
4-5 quarts water
2 large onions, peeled and quartered
3 carrots, rinsed and chopped
2 stalks celery plus leaves, rinsed and chopped
2–3 cloves garlic, peeled
5 to 6 sprigs fresh thyme leaves or 1 teaspoon dried
2 bay leaves
½ bunch fresh parsley with stems

Preparation

1. Preheat oven to 400°F.

2. Place the bones on a rimmed baking sheet. Roast 20-30 minutes.

3. Transfer the bones to an 8-quart stockpot, and add 4-5 quarts water, the onions, carrots, celery, and garlic.

4. Bring to a boil, skim off and discard any foam or scum that rises to the top.

5. Add thyme and bay leaves.

6. Reduce heat to low. Cover, and simmer 8-12 hours or longer. The longer you cook stock, the more concentrated it becomes. During the last hour of cooking, add the parsley.

7. Strain the stock into containers; discard the bones and vegetables.

8. Pour into jars and store in the refrigerator overnight.

9. Skim and discard fat.

If freezing stock, leave 1 to 2 inches of empty space inside the container for expansion as the stock expands as it freezes. You can freeze stock for 3-4 months.

BREAKFAST OPTIONS

People often get stuck in a breakfast rut. If they are not pouring cold milk onto boxed cereal flakes, they simply have no idea what to eat. In this section, I've included many breakfast options that are easy and delicious and can benefit the health of your thyroid as well as the rest of your beautiful body.

It doesn't take much effort to prepare a nourishing breakfast; it just takes the desire to eat well and support your body. Try a new breakfast choice every day, and see which foods your body likes best.

Porridge

Porridge is cereal grains prepared with water or milk and cooked until thick, creamy, and delicious. Softening and cooking grains renders them more digestible. I used rice in this recipe, but any grain can be used to make porridge: corn, wheat, rye, quinoa, amaranth, millet, rice, barley, spelt, kamut, buckwheat, and farro. This recipe also works well with any leftover grain. If you have a gluten allergy, do not use wheat, rye, spelt, kamut, or farro.

Ingredients

1 cup cooked brown rice
2 cups water or milk
1–2 tablespoons raisins
1 or 2 dashes ground cinnamon
¼ cup walnuts, dry roasted and crushed

2 to 3 tablespoons yogurt, kefir, or cream

Preparation

1. In a medium pot, bring rice, water, raisins, and cinnamon to a boil.

2. Reduce heat to medium.

3. Cover and cook until creamy, 7 to 10 minutes.

4. Remove from heat, and transfer to individual bowls.

5. Serve hot, topped with walnuts and yogurt.

Soaking and Roasting Nuts and Seeds

Ingredients

Shelled walnuts, almonds, pecans, hazelnuts, filberts, pistachios
Pumpkin, sunflower, chia, sesame, and flax seeds (do NOT roast flax seeds, only soak them)
Sea salt

Preparation

1. Soak nuts or seeds 8-10 hours in room temperature water.

2. Preheat oven to 125°F–175°F (maximum 175°F). Some ovens don't have low temperatures. If that's the case with your oven, put it on the "warm" setting, or put it on the lowest setting and leave the oven door open a crack to reduce the internal temperature.

3. Discard soaking water, and place nuts onto a rimmed baking sheet.

4. Season with sea salt.

5. Roast nuts in the oven until lightly browned and dry, 2-6 hours.

6. Roast seeds until dry, a shorter duration of 1-3 hours.

Congee

This breakfast dish is a traditional grain porridge eaten in many cultures around the world. This recipe needs to be started the night before.

Ingredients

1 cup whole grain brown rice, soaked overnight in water to cover
5 cups water or milk
1 teaspoon sea salt

Preparation

1. Drain rice, and discard soaking water.

2. Place rice and water in a medium pot and bring to a boil.

3. Add salt, cover, and reduce heat to simmer.

4. Cook 2 to 3 hours, or until you get a soupy consistency.

5. Additions: During the last ½ hour of cooking, you can add ingredients:
   Tofu, Meat, Fish, Vegetables, Seaweed, Nuts, Fruits
   Anything you think would be enjoyable in your version of congee

Miso Salmon Soup

Soup for breakfast? Yes! This is a great way to start the day. Soup is warming and gentle on the digestive system.

I especially love soups in the wintertime, or anytime it's cold outside. I certainly have enjoyed this soup all year round by switching up the ingredients as the seasons change.

Ingredients

1 small onion, peeled and cut into thin crescents
2-3 shitake mushrooms, thinly sliced
4 cups water or fish stock
3 to 4 ounces salmon or other fish
2-3 leaves bok choy or other leafy greens, cut into bite–size pieces
3-4 tablespoon sweet miso
2-3 scallions, white and light green parts, minced

Preparation

1. Place onions, mushrooms, and water in a medium pot; bring to a boil.

2. Reduce heat to low.

3. Add fish and bok choy, and simmer, covered, 3–5 minutes.

4. In a small bowl, dilute miso in a small amount of the cooking water from the soup pot, and stir back into the soup.

5. Continue simmering for 2–3 minutes.

6. Ladle into individual bowls. Serve garnished with scallions.

Oats and Almonds with Dried Berries

Rolled oats are quick cooking and contain less phytic acid than cracked oats, steel cut oats, and whole oat groats. Rolled oats have already been steamed and pressed. You could soak rolled oats overnight, but generally you do not need to.

I used goji berries in this recipe. If you have a reaction to "nightshades," then swap out the goji berries for dried cranberries, blueberries, or any other berries you prefer.

Ingredients

¼ teaspoon sea salt
¼ cup dried goji berries
1 dash ground cinnamon
1 dash ground nutmeg
1 cup rolled oats
¼ cup slivered almonds, (soaked, blanched, and/or roasted)
¼ cup yogurt, kefir, or milk

Preparation

1. Place 2 cups water, the salt, berries, cinnamon, nutmeg, and oats in a medium pot. Bring to a boil.

2. Cover pot, reduce heat to low, and cook until oats thicken, 7–10 minutes.

3. Ladle into individual bowls.

4. Serve topped with almonds and yogurt.

Savory Oats and Sausage

Many people begin their days with sweet oats or other sweetened cereal grains. This recipe is for all of the folks who like more savory foods.

Ingredients

1 cup rolled oats
1 tablespoon grass-fed butter
1 pinch sea salt
¼ teaspoon ground cinnamon and/or ground cardamom
⅛ teaspoon ground nutmeg (optional)
2 teaspoons olive oil or other fat
2 pork, chicken, or turkey sausage links, diced
1 tablespoon sauerkraut or other type of pickled food per serving
Parsley leaves, minced

Preparation

1. Place 2 cups water, the oats, butter, salt, cinnamon, and nutmeg in a medium pot. Bring to a boil.

2. Reduce heat to low. Cover, and cook 6-8 minutes.

3. While oats are cooking, heat oil in a skillet over medium-high heat.

4. Add sausages, and cook until done, 8-10 minutes.

5. Place oats into individual bowls, approximately ½ cup per person.

6. Top oats with sausages.

7. Serve garnished with 1 tablespoon sauerkraut and some minced parsley.

Rolled Oats with Fresh Fruit and Seeds

Ingredients

½ cup rolled oats

1 pinch sea salt

½ apple or pear, cored and diced (in the winter) OR ¼ cup fresh blueberries or blackberries (in the summer)

⅓ cup whole milk, coconut milk, oat milk, or any other milk

¼ cup sunflower or other seeds, roasted

Preparation

1. Place 1½ cups water and the oats in a medium pot; bring to a boil.

2. Add salt.

3. During the cold months, cook the heartier fruit of apple or pear, with the oats over medium heat for 7-10 minutes.

4. In the warmer months, cook the oats 7-10 minutes, and then top them with the berries at the end of cooking.

5. At the end of cooking, stir in your favorite milk.

6. Serve, garnished with crunchy toasted seeds.

Poached Eggs

Ingredients

1 tablespoon apple cider vinegar
1 or 2 eggs per person
Sourdough bread, 1 slice per person
Grass-fed butter
Sea salt
Freshly ground black pepper

Preparation

1. In a small pot, bring 2-3 cups water to a boil. Add vinegar.

2. Reduce heat to medium-low.

3. Crack egg(s) into a small bowl and then gently slide egg(s) into the water. Don't crowd the pot. I generally cook 1-2 eggs at a time.

4. Cook 4 minutes for a soft egg or 5 minutes for a firmer egg.

5. While eggs are cooking, put bread into the toaster. Butter toast and place it on a plate.

6. Use a slotted spoon to gently lift egg from the water. Set the egg onto a paper towel to dry.

7. Place egg on top of buttered toast, and sprinkle with salt and pepper.

8. Repeat with other eggs.

Creamy Polenta and Fried Eggs

Ingredients

½ cup polenta (corn meal)
Sea salt
2 tablespoons grass-fed butter
Ghee, coconut oil, or olive oil
1–2 eggs per person
Freshly ground black pepper
Hot sauce
Parsley leaves, minced

Preparation

1. In a medium pot, bring 1¾ cups water to a boil.

2. Add polenta, ¼ teaspoon salt, and butter.

3. Reduce heat to low. Simmer, stirring frequently, until polenta is thick and creamy, about 15-20 minutes. Transfer to individual bowls.

4. In a skillet, heat ghee over medium heat.

5. Crack eggs into the pan—try to keep the yolks intact.

6. Sprinkle 1 pinch each salt and pepper on top of each egg.

7. Cook eggs until lightly crispy around the edges.

8. Top each bowl of polenta with a fried egg.

9. Top each egg with a dash of hot sauce and some parsley.

Buckwheat with Poached Eggs

Cream of buckwheat is milled buckwheat and can be found at most health food stores. Buckwheat is gluten-free.

Ingredients

2½ cups water or milk
2 tablespoons grass-fed butter
Sea salt
½ cup cream of buckwheat
1 tablespoon apple cider vinegar
1–2 eggs per serving
Freshly ground black pepper
1 tablespoon sauerkraut per serving

Preparation

1. In a medium pot, bring water to a boil.
2. Add butter, 1-2 pinches salt, and the buckwheat.
3. Reduce heat to low.
4. Cover and simmer 8-10 minutes. Spoon into individual bowls.
5. Pour 2-3 cups water into a small pot. Bring to a boil, and add 1 tablespoon vinegar.
6. Crack open eggs and slide into the water without breaking the yolk.
7. Cook 4 minutes for a soft egg, 5 minutes for a firmer egg.
8. Transfer eggs to a paper towel to drain.
9. Place an egg on top of cooked buckwheat. Season with salt and pepper.
10. Top each egg with 1 tablespoon sauerkraut.

Scrambled Eggs with Vegetables

Ingredients

¼ cup broccoli florets per person
2 tablespoons grass-fed butter or olive oil
2 scallions, white and light green parts, minced
Sea salt
2 eggs per person, beaten
¼ cup grated raw milk Cheddar cheese (optional)
Freshly ground black pepper

Preparation

1. Pour ¼ cup water into a small frying pan. Bring to a boil.

2. Place broccoli florets into the water and cook until bright green and the water has evaporated, 1-2 minutes.

3. Add butter and scallions and a few pinches of sea salt.

4. Reduce heat to medium-low.

5. Add beaten eggs, and use a wooden spoon or spatula to pull the eggs away from the sides of the pan.

6. Continue pulling the eggs from the sides of the pan to the center until the eggs are firm but still moist.

7. Serve topped with cheese and pepper.

Variations of Scrambled Eggs with Vegetables:

8. Add sautéed chopped red bell pepper and chopped onions with the broccoli and scallions.

9. Add sautéed chopped leeks and sliced mushrooms with the broccoli and scallions.

10. Serve garnished with minced chives or other fresh herbs.

Root Hash with Poached Eggs

For those of you who don't eat grains, try this delicious root hash as a bed for your eggs. You can switch up the roots and try it with tubers like potatoes, too.

Ingredients

1 parsnip (or other root), rinsed
1 medium beet, rinsed
2-3 carrots, rinsed
2 scallions, white and light green parts, rinsed and minced
Sea salt
1 tablespoon fresh thyme leaves or 1 teaspoon dried
2-3 tablespoons grass-fed butter
Fresh eggs
1 tablespoon apple cider vinegar
Freshly ground black pepper

Preparation

For the Root Hash
1. Rinse parsnip, beet, and carrots.
2. Use a food processor or a cheese grater to shred the vegetables into a bowl.
3. Add scallions, and season with ¼ teaspoon sea salt and the thyme.
4. Let the veggies sit for a few minutes, and then squeeze them to release any excess water.
5. Heat a frying pan and add butter.
6. Form hash into round palm-sized ½-inch thick patties
7. Cook patties until golden, 7-10 minutes on each side.
8. Taste, and season with more salt if needed.

For the Poached Eggs
1. Bring 2-3 cups water to a boil in a small saucepot.
2. Reduce heat to low.
3. Add 1 tablespoon vinegar to the water.
4. Crack an egg and gently slide it into the water.
5. Cook 4 minutes for a soft egg, 5 minutes for a firmer egg.
6. Remove egg with a slotted spoon, and lay on a paper towel to absorb the water.
7. Lay cooked egg on top of Root Hash patty.
8. Season with salt and pepper.

GRAINS

Often, I'll hear from folks who are on a no-grain diet. They tell me they felt great in the beginning. After a few months, their energy levels crashed or they developed a thyroid condition, and they don't understand why.

Grains have been part of the human food supply for thousands of years. I would suggest you think twice before cutting them completely from your diet. Try some of these delicious recipes and see how your body reacts. That'll be the best indicator of whether this type of food is working for you. Most of these recipes already have a small amount of animal protein included, or are made with stock, which would make them basically a one-pot meal.

Jumpin' Jambalaya

Ingredients

1 tablespoon olive oil

1 large onion, peeled and diced

3 cloves garlic, peeled and minced

2 stalks celery, rinsed and diced

2 carrots, rinsed and diced

1 red pepper, rinsed, seeded, and diced

1 (15-ounce) can crushed tomatoes, undrained

1 cup long grain brown rice, soaked overnight in water to cover

1 (12-ounce) package Andouille turkey or chicken sausages,
   cut into ½-inch rounds

1-2 teaspoons hot sauce

2 tablespoons minced fresh thyme leaves or 2 teaspoons dried

1 teaspoon sea salt

½ teaspoon freshly ground black pepper

2 cups water or chicken stock

1 pound shrimp, peeled and deveined

3 tablespoons minced fresh parsley leaves

Preparation

1. Heat oil in a large soup pot over medium-high heat.
   Add onions, garlic, and celery, and cook 3-5 minutes.

2. Add carrots, peppers, tomatoes, rice, sausages, hot sauce, thyme, salt, pepper, and water.

3. Cover and bring to a boil.

4. Reduce heat to low. Cover, and cook 35 minutes.

5. Add shrimp and parsley.

6. Cover, and continue cooking 7-10 minutes.

7. With a large spoon, mix all ingredients (from the bottom of the pot to the top of the pot, to incorporate the shrimp) before serving.

Quick-Cooking Fried Rice

Ingredients

1 onion, peeled and diced
2 cloves garlic, peeled and minced
½ cup broccoli or cauliflower florets, rinsed
1 carrot, rinsed and diced
½ teaspoon sea salt
1 tablespoon peanut oil
2-3 eggs, beaten
1 cup cooked brown rice
1 tablespoon toasted sesame oil
2-3 tablespoons tamari
1 tablespoon mirin rice wine (optional)
2 scallions, white and light green parts, minced

Preparation

1. Place ¼-⅓ cup water into a large sauté pan and bring to a boil. Add the onions, garlic, broccoli, and carrots; water sauté, 3-5 minutes or until water evaporates.

2. Add salt.

3. In a separate pan, heat oil over medium heat. Add eggs and scramble. Chop into bite-size pieces.

4. Stir the cooked eggs and the rice into the pan with the vegetables.

5. Season with sesame oil, tamari, and mirin.

6. Toss, and cook an additional 3-5 minutes.

7. Serve garnished with scallions.

Polenta with Sautéed Wild Mushrooms and Greens

Ingredients

6 cups water, chicken stock, or vegetable stock
2 cups finely ground cornmeal (polenta)
1½ teaspoons sea salt, divided
1 tablespoon grass-fed butter or olive oil
1 large onion, peeled and cut into thin crescents
8-10 shitake mushrooms, stems removed, thinly sliced
1 ounce maitake mushrooms, chopped
½ pound ground turkey or pork (optional)
2 cups chopped greens (bok choy, collards, dandelion, etc.), rinsed
½ cup diced fresh tomatoes
2 tablespoons fresh thyme leaves
¼ cup shredded raw milk cheese, (optional)

Preparation

1. Combine water and cornmeal in a saucepan. Bring to a boil.

2. Reduce heat to medium-low.

3. Add 1 teaspoon salt. Cook uncovered, stirring occasionally to prevent lumps. Set aside.

4. Heat butter over medium heat in a frying pan,
    Add onions and sauté for 1-2 minutes.

5. Add mushrooms and continue cooking 2-3 minutes.

6. Add ground meat, and break into small pieces as it cooks.

7. Add greens, tomatoes, remaining ½ teaspoon salt, and the thyme.

8. Continue cooking until greens are soft, 5-7 minutes.

9. Pour cooked cornmeal (polenta) into a 9- ×13-inch casserole dish. Let set 10-12 minutes.

10. Top polenta with the mushrooms, vegetables, and meat.

11. Cut the polenta into squares and serve, garnished with shredded cheese.

Quinoa and Black-Eyed Pea Salad with Smoked Chimichurri Dressing

Ingredients

1 cup organic red or white quinoa, soaked in water to cover,
  5-6 hours or overnight
2 inches dried kelp
¼ teaspoon sea salt
1½ cups cooked black-eyed peas, or 1 (15-ounce) can black-eyed peas, rinsed
1 bell pepper, rinsed, seeded, and diced
1 shallot, peeled and minced

Chimichurri Dressing

1½ cups cilantro, (or 1 bunch), rinsed
3 cloves garlic, peeled
2 tablespoons fresh oregano leaves or 2 teaspoons dried
½ teaspoon smoked paprika
½ cup extra virgin olive oil
2 tablespoons white wine vinegar
Juice of 1 lime
1 teaspoon sea salt
Butter lettuce leaves (or other lettuce), rinsed, to use as cups

Preparation

1. Drain quinoa and discard soaking water.

2. Place quinoa, kelp, and 1¾ cups water into a pot.

3. Bring to a boil. Cover, season with salt, and reduce heat to low.

4. Cook until liquid evaporates, 12-15 minutes.

5. In a large mixing bowl, combine quinoa, black-eyed peas, peppers, and shallots.

6. Puree the Chimichurri Dressing ingredients in a food processor.

7. Mix Chimichurri Dressing into the salad.

8. Spoon the mixture into lettuce cups.

Kasha Pilaf with Maitake Mushrooms

Ingredients

2 tablespoons grass-fed butter

3 shallots, peeled and minced

2 stalks celery, rinsed and diced

1 carrot, rinsed and diced

½ cup chopped fresh maitake mushrooms or ¼ cup dried maitake
   (soaked in room temperature water)

1 teaspoon dried thyme leaves or 1 tablespoon fresh

½ teaspoon sea salt

2 cups chicken stock, veggie stock, or water

1 cup kasha (toasted buckwheat)

Fresh parsley leaves

Preparation

1. Heat butter in a deep frying pan over medium heat. Add shallots and sauté for 2-3 minutes.

2. Add celery, carrots, and mushrooms.

3. Cover, and continue cooking 3-5 minutes.

4. Add thyme, salt, and stock; bring to a boil.

5. Add kasha and bring back up to a boil.

6. Cover, and reduce heat to simmer.

7. Cook until all the liquid has cooked off, 12-15 minutes.

8. Fluff with a fork, and serve garnished with fresh parsley.

Quick-Cooking Quinoa and Lamb Salad

Ingredients

2 cups organic quinoa, soaked for 3-5 hours or overnight in water to cover
3¼ cups vegetable stock or water
Sea salt
1 (6-10 ounce) grass-fed lamb steak
¼ teaspoon ground cumin
¼ teaspoon freshly ground black pepper
¼ teaspoon ground cinnamon
⅓ cup plus 1 tablespoon extra virgin olive oil
1 red and 1 yellow bell pepper, rinsed, seeded, and diced
5-6 leaves fresh basil, thinly sliced
¼ cup fresh mint leaves, thinly sliced
2-3 tablespoons minced fresh parsley leaves
2-3 tablespoons white wine vinegar

Preparation

1. Drain quinoa, and discard soaking water.

2. Place quinoa and stock into a soup pot. Bring to a boil.

3. Add ¼ teaspoon salt.

4. Cover, reduce heat to low, and simmer until liquid is fully absorbed, 10-12 minutes. Set aside to cool.

5. Chop lamb steak into 1-inch bite-size pieces.

6. Season lamb with cumin, salt, pepper, and cinnamon.

7. Heat 1 tablespoon oil in a frying pan. Add lamb, and cook 2-3 minutes per side.

8. Remove lamb from frying pan, and let rest on a plate for 3-5 minutes.

9. In a large mixing bowl, combine quinoa, peppers, basil, mint, parsley, and lamb.

10. Whisk the remaining ⅓ cup oil with vinegar in a small bowl. Season with salt and pepper to taste.

11. Toss quinoa and lamb salad with the dressing.

BEANS

Beans are a great source of vegetable protein and dietary fiber, plus starch for energy. As long as they are prepared properly (soaked and cooked with salt), they can be a good addition to a thyroid-supportive diet. Just don't eat mountains of beans! And, make sure you exercise or move your body in some way to help burn off that starch (sugar) and move the fiber through your system.

If you have blood sugar issues, you may feel sleepy after eating plain beans, or any starchy foods in excess. Preparing beans with a small amount of fat and/or animal protein can help slow sugar absorption.

Black-Eyed Peas with Chorizo

Ingredients

1½ cups black-eyed peas, soaked overnight in water to cover, or 2 (15-ounce) cans, rinsed and drained
2 bay leaves
1½ teaspoons sea salt, divided
1 tablespoon olive oil
2 onions, peeled and diced
5 cloves garlic, peeled and minced
3-4 ounces chorizo or other sausage, diced
1½ cups chicken stock or water
1 tablespoon fresh oregano leaves or 1 teaspoon dried
Freshly ground black pepper
1 tablespoon minced fresh parsley leaves

Preparation

1. Drain black-eyed peas and discard soaking water. Place beans in a medium pot. (If using canned beans, start at #6)

2. Add 3 cups water and bring peas to a boil.

3. Skim and discard foam that rises to the top.

4. Add bay leaves, cover, and simmer over low heat for 30 minutes.

5. Add 1 teaspoon salt, and continue cooking until beans are soft, about 15 minutes. If there is any liquid left, drain the beans.

6. Heat oil in a deep frying pan over medium heat. Add onions and garlic, and sauté 2-3 minutes.

7. Add chorizo and cook until done, 5-7 minutes.

8. Add beans, stock, and oregano.

9. Season with pepper and remaining ½ teaspoon salt. Adjust to taste.

10. Cover, and cook over medium-low heat for 10 minutes.

11. Remove and discard the bay leaves.

12. Serve garnished with fresh parsley.

Savory Lentil and Vegetable Stew with Crispy Kale Chips

Ingredients

1 cup lentils, soaked overnight in water to cover
5 cups water or chicken stock
2 inches dried alaria or kelp sea vegetable
1 tablespoon olive oil
1 leek, white and light green parts, cleaned and cut into 1-inch pieces
2-3 cloves garlic, peeled and minced
2 parsnips, rinsed and diced into ½-inch pieces
3 carrots, rinsed and diced into ½-inch pieces
½ cup celeriac (celery root), rinsed, peeled, and diced into ½-inch cubes
1 potato, diced into ½-inch cubes
1 tablespoon fresh thyme leaves or 1 teaspoon dried
1½ teaspoons sea salt
¼ teaspoon freshly ground black pepper
Crispy Kale Chips (see recipe on the next page)

Preparation

1. Drain lentils and discard soaking water.

2. Place lentils and water in a soup pot; bring to a boil. Reduce heat to low. Cover, and simmer 35 minutes.

3. Add alaria, oil, leeks, garlic, parsnips, carrots, celeriac, potatoes, thyme, salt, and pepper.

4. Cover, and bring back up to a boil.

5. Reduce heat to medium-low, and cook 20-25 minutes.

6. Remove one-third of the ingredients, and puree them in a food processor or blender.

7. Return the puree to the soup.

8. Serve garnished with Crispy Kale Chips.

Crispy Kale Chips

Ingredients

1 bunch kale, rinsed and dried
1 tablespoon olive oil
Sea salt

Preparation

1. Preheat oven to 350°F.

2. Remove kale stems (can discard or save for stir fry).

3. Rip kale leaves into bite-size pieces and place into a large bowl.

4. Season with oil. Do NOT add salt.

5. Place oiled kale onto a cookie sheet or baking tray.

6. Roast until kale is crispy, 10-12 minutes.

7. Remove from the oven, and season lightly with salt.

Spicy Black Bean Soup with Polenta Croutons

Ingredients

1 tablespoon olive oil
1 large onion, peeled and diced
3 cloves garlic, peeled and minced
1½ teaspoons ground cumin
1 carrot, rinsed and diced
2 stalks celery, rinsed and diced
1 red bell pepper, rinsed, seeded, and diced
1 jalapeño pepper, rinsed, seeded, and diced
2 cups cooked black beans, or 2 cups rinsed and drained canned beans
4 cups veggie stock, chicken stock, or water
1 teaspoon sea salt
¼ cup chopped fresh cilantro leaves

Preparation

1. Heat oil in a skillet over medium heat. Add onions, garlic, and cumin, and sauté 1-2 minutes.

2. Add carrots, celery, bell peppers, jalapeños, beans, and stock.

3. Bring to a boil; add salt. Cover, and simmer over medium-low heat 10-15 minutes.

4. Stir cilantro into the pot at the end of cooking.

Polenta Croutons

Ingredients

Sea salt

1 cup polenta or corn grits

1-2 tablespoons grass-fed butter

3-4 tablespoons coconut oil

Preparation

1. Pour 2¾ cups water into a medium pot. Bring to a boil; stir in 1 teaspoon salt, polenta, and butter.

2. Lower heat to simmer.

3. Cook, stirring frequently, until the polenta thickens, 15-20 minutes.

4. Pour polenta into a 9-inch square baking dish, and let set for 45 minutes at room temperature.

5. Cut the polenta into 4 equal sections.

6. Remove one of the sections and dice it into one-inch cubes.

7. In a frying pan, heat oil.

8. Drop cubes into the hot oil, and fry until light brown and crispy on all sides.

9. Transfer to paper towels to drain. Sprinkle with salt.

10. Repeat with remaining polenta, or refrigerate the polenta and fry up large squares for a fun breakfast treat with eggs.

Creamy Cannellini Beans and Kale Soup

Ingredients

1½ cups cannellini beans, soaked overnight in water to cover
3-4 inches dried kelp
2 bay leaves
1 teaspoon sea salt
2 tablespoons olive oil
1 onion, peeled and diced
3 cloves garlic, peeled and minced
4-5 kale leaves, rinsed, dried, and chopped
4 cups water, vegetable stock, or chicken stock
1/4 teaspoon dried rosemary leaves
1 teaspoon dried thyme leaves
Sea salt
Freshly ground black pepper

Preparation

1. Drain beans and discard soaking water. Place beans, kelp, and 3 cups water in a medium pot. Bring to a boil.

2. Skim off and discard any foam that rises to the top.

3. Add bay leaves, cover, and lower heat to low. Simmer 1 hour and 15 minutes.

4. Add salt, and continue cooking 15-20 minutes.

5. Heat oil in a soup pot over medium-high heat. Add onions and garlic; sauté 2-3 minutes.

6. Add kale and cook until wilted.

7. Add water, rosemary, and thyme.

8. Remove and discard the bay leaves.

9. Puree half the cooked beans in a food processor to achieve a creamy consistency. Add all of the beans to the soup. Bring to a boil.

10. Lower heat to medium, season with salt and pepper, and cook an additional 5-7 minutes.

ANIMAL PROTEINS

Animal meats, fats, and bones are traditional foods containing vital nutrients that can benefit the muscles, heart, and endocrine system. People suffering from adrenal fatigue and thyroid disease may need to increase the amount and types of proteins they are eating, as well as improve the way those proteins are cooked.

For example, someone suffering from a weak digestive system may need proteins that are braised for long periods of time, breaking down the muscle fibers and making the meat easier to digest.

Animal proteins that would be better for someone feeling cold are generally the warming red meats instead of the more cooling fish. If someone is hot, fish would be the better option.

There are lots of recipes for you to experiment with. Try to find a healthful balance of white meat, red meat, and fish to discover what works best for your system and for your condition.

Braised Lamb Shanks

Ingredients

3-4 small pastured lamb shanks (or 1 per person)
Sea salt
Freshly ground black pepper
Ground cumin
Ground cinnamon
2 tablespoons pork fat or other fat or oil (can use peanut oil or coconut oil)
2 cups red wine
4-5 cups beef, chicken, vegetable stock, or water (enough to cover shanks)
2 bay leaves
2 onions, peeled and quartered
2-3 stalks celery, rinsed and chopped
2-3 carrots, rinsed and chopped
2 tablespoons fresh rosemary leaves
3-4 sprigs fresh thyme leaves
1 teaspoon sea salt
4-6 cloves garlic, peeled and chopped
8-10 fingerling potatoes, rinsed

Preparation

1. Season shanks with equal parts salt, pepper, cumin, and cinnamon.
2. Heat fat in a large deep frying pan, and sear shanks until lightly browned on all sides.
3. Add wine and enough stock to cover shanks.
4. Bring to a boil. Cover, and reduce heat to low.
5. Cook 1 hour and 45 minutes.
6. Uncover, and turn the shanks with tongs.
7. Add bay leaves, onions, celery, carrots, rosemary, thyme, salt, garlic, and potatoes.
8. Replace cover, and continue cooking another 1½ hours (3-3½ hours total cooking time).
9. Transfer shanks and vegetables to a serving plate.
10. Cook the broth (jus) over high heat until reduced by half.
11. Remove and discard thyme sprigs and bay leaves.
12. Drizzle reduced jus on top of shanks.

Hearty Grass-Fed Beef Stew with Vegetables

Ingredients

¾ pound grass-fed beef chuck, cubed
Ground cumin
Freshly ground black pepper
1 teaspoon sea salt
1 tablespoon peanut oil
1 tablespoon olive oil
1 onion, peeled and chopped
4 cloves garlic, peeled and minced
1 small celeriac (celery root), peeled and chopped or 2-3 stalks celery, rinsed and diced
2 carrots, rinsed and chopped
2 red potatoes, rinsed and chopped
2 bay leaves
4 cups beef stock or water
Sea salt
Fresh parsley leaves, minced

Preparation

1. Season meat with cumin, pepper, and salt.

2. Heat peanut oil in a frying pan over medium heat.

3. Add meat and sauté until lightly browned on all sides.

4. Cover, and cook 5-7 minutes.

5. Heat olive oil in a soup pot over medium heat.
   Add onions and garlic, and sauté for 2-3minutes.

6. Add celeriac, carrots, and potatoes, and cook 2-3 minutes.

7. Add the pan-seared meat plus its juices to the soup pot.

8. Add bay leaves, stock, and salt to taste.

9. Bring to a boil.

10. Cover and reduce heat to low.

11. Simmer 45 minutes to 1 hour.

12. Remove and discard the bay leaves.

13. Serve garnished with parsley.

Sautéed Shallots and Chicken Livers

Ingredients

2 tablespoons grass-fed or organic butter
2-3 shallots, peeled and minced
1 tablespoon fresh thyme leaves or 1 teaspoon dried
¼ cup mirin rice wine (can use any sweet white wine)
3-4 chicken livers, cleaned and chopped
½ cup chicken stock or water
Sea salt
Freshly ground black pepper
Fresh parsley leaves

Preparation

1. Heat butter in a frying pan over medium-low heat.
   Add shallots and thyme, and sauté until wilted, 2-3 minutes.

2. Add mirin, chicken livers, and stock.
   Season with pinches of salt and pepper.

3. Cook until liquid evaporates.

4. Serve garnished with fresh parsley.

Gluten-Free Creamy Turkey Chowder

Ingredients

2 tablespoons grass-fed or organic butter

2-3 tablespoons white rice flour or other flour

4 cups turkey or chicken stock or water

1 leek, white and light green parts, cleaned and chopped

1 tablespoon minced fresh sage leaves

1 teaspoon minced fresh rosemary leaves

2 to 3 cloves garlic, peeled and minced

½ cup celeriac (celery root), peeled and diced, or 2 stalks celery, rinsed and diced

2 carrots, rinsed and diced

1 medium-sized potato, rinsed and diced

1 teaspoon sea salt

Freshly ground black pepper

1½ cups cubed cooked turkey

1 tablespoon minced fresh parsley leaves

Preparation

1. Whisk together butter and flour in a soup pot over medium-low heat.

2. Add stock gradually, whisking continually so the flour doesn't clump. Whisk until smooth.

3. Add leeks, sage, rosemary, garlic, celeriac, carrots, potatoes, and salt. Season with pepper.

4. Cover and bring to a boil. Reduce heat to medium, and cook 15-18 minutes.

5. Add turkey, mix, and cook 3-5 minutes.

6. Adjust seasoning to taste. Serve garnished with parsley.

Old-Fashioned Chicken Soup

Ingredients

5 cups chicken stock or water
1 teaspoon dried thyme leaves
2 onions, peeled and diced
3-4 stalks celery, rinsed and diced
2-3 carrots, rinsed and cut into thin rounds
2 red potatoes, rinsed and diced (can use other potatoes)
Organic/pastured chicken wings and drumsticks from one chicken
2 teaspoons sea salt
¼ cup chopped fresh parsley leaves
2-3 cloves garlic, peeled and minced

Preparation

1. Place stock, thyme, onions, celery, carrots, potatoes, chicken, and salt in a soup pot. Bring to a boil.

2. Reduce heat to low, cover, and simmer for 40-45 minutes.

3. Stir in parsley and garlic, and continue cooking 3-5 minutes.

Grilled Teriyaki Salmon

Ingredients

1 pound wild salmon
¼ cup shoyu or wheat-free tamari
1 tablespoon maple syrup
2 tablespoons apple cider vinegar
2 cloves garlic, peeled and minced
1 tablespoon peeled and minced ginger
Coconut oil or other high heat oil for brushing
2-3 scallions, white and light green parts, rinsed and minced

Preparation

1. Place salmon in a flat container or baking dish.

2. In a small bowl, combine shoyu, maple syrup, vinegar, garlic, ginger, and ⅓ cup water, and pour over salmon.

3. Cover and marinate 25-35 minutes at room temperature or in the refrigerator overnight. The longer you marinate in the liquid, the more flavor infuses into the fish.

4. Brush your grill pan with oil.

5. Transfer salmon to the grill pan (or outside on an actual grill), and cook for 3-5 minutes per side, depending on the thickness of the fish (a total of 10 minutes per inch of thickness).

6. Serve garnished with scallions.

Bone-Building Salmon Salad

Ingredients

1 (7.5-ounce) can wild salmon—preferably with bones and skin, drained
1 small red onion, peeled and minced
1 celery stalk, rinsed and diced small
⅓ cup extra virgin olive oil
1 teaspoon prepared Dijon mustard
1-2 teaspoons local honey
2-3 tablespoons apple cider vinegar
Sea salt
Freshly ground black pepper
Sourdough bread or Romaine lettuce

Preparation

1. Place salmon in a mixing bowl and mash with a fork.

2. Add onions and celery.

3. In a small bowl, whisk together oil, mustard, honey, and vinegar.

4. Season with salt and pepper to taste.

5. Combine dressing with salmon and mix thoroughly.

6. Enjoy on sourdough bread or wrap in Romaine lettuce.

Steamed Mussels with Mirin

Ingredients

2 pounds mussels
Sea salt
1 tablespoon flour or cornmeal
1 link chorizo sausage, diced
3-4 shallots, peeled and thinly sliced
3 cloves garlic, peeled and minced
½ cup mirin rice wine or 1 cup white wine
¼ bulb fennel, rinsed and thinly sliced
Few sprigs of fresh parsley leaves, chopped
¼ cup chopped cilantro
1 tablespoon grass-fed butter

Preparation

1. Place mussels into a large bowl with 4 cups water, the salt, and flour. The flour helps the mussels purge any sand.

2. Keep mussels submerged for 1 hour.

3. Discard the water and rinse the mussels in fresh water. Discard any mussels that have broken shells or a bad smell.

4. In a soup pot, sauté chorizo until it releases most of its fat.

5. Add the shallots and garlic, and sauté 2-3 minutes.

6. Add mirin and fennel, and cook 2-3 minutes.

7. Add the mussels to the pot. Cover and cook 5-6 minutes. Discard any mussels that are still closed; they are not edible.

8. Add parsley, cilantro, and butter.

9. Taste the liquid before salting. The mussels will release a briny salty liquid. Do not oversalt.

Savory Mushroom and Herb Frittata

Ingredients

1 tablespoon olive oil

1 medium onion, peeled and sliced into thin half moons

5-6 shitake mushrooms, wiped with a damp towel or brushed, thinly sliced
(discard the stems or save the stems for stock)

5-6 cremini mushrooms, thinly sliced

1 tablespoon fresh thyme leaves or ½ teaspoon dried

1 tablespoon fresh tarragon leaves or ½ teaspoon dried

¼ teaspoon sea salt

2-3 tablespoons grass-fed butter

7-8 eggs, beaten

Fresh chives, minced

Preparation

1. Preheat oven to 350°F.

2. Heat oil in an ovenproof frying pan over medium heat. Add onions and
   mushrooms. Sauté until the onions are translucent and mushrooms are
   wilted, 5-7 minutes.

3. Add thyme, tarragon, salt, and butter.

4. After the butter melts, add the eggs.

5. Cook on the stovetop 2-3 minutes or until eggs begin to set.

6. Remove the pan from the stovetop and place into the oven until eggs
   fluff up, 10-12 minutes.

7. Serve garnished with minced chives.

Sea Bass Soup with Soba Noodles

Ingredients

1 (8 or 9-ounce) package soba noodles
5 cups fish stock or water
1 leek, white and light green parts, cleaned and cut in thick diagonals
2 inches ginger, peeled and cut into thin matchsticks
1 cup chopped Chinese cabbage
1 carrot, rinsed and cut into ¼-inch thick diagonals
12-16 ounces black sea bass or black cod, with skin, cut into four equal pieces (1 piece per serving)
4 tablespoons sweet white miso
1 sheet toasted nori, cut into thin slivers

Preparation

1. Bring a large pot of water to a boil. Add soba noodles, and cook according to directions on package.

2. Drain and set aside.

3. While noodles are cooking, in a separate pot, bring stock, leeks, ginger, cabbage, and carrots to a boil.

4. Reduce heat to low, and cook 5-7 minutes.

5. Add fish, cover, and cook 3 minutes.

6. In a small bowl, dilute miso with a ladle of liquid from the soup, and stir back into the soup.

7. Reduce heat to very low, cover, and simmer 3-4 minutes.

8. For each serving, place a portion of noodles in the bottom of a bowl, and ladle soup and one piece of fish on top.

9. Serve garnished with slivers of toasted nori.

Creamy Oyster Chowder

Rich in zinc, iodine, and B12, this oyster chowder is sure to please your palate as well as your thyroid.

Ingredients

1 tablespoon olive oil
1 onion, peeled and diced
2 medium Yukon Gold potatoes, peeled and diced
5 cups chicken stock
2 stalks celery, rinsed and diced
2 carrots, rinsed and diced
1½ teaspoons fresh tarragon leaves or ½ teaspoon dried
1 teaspoon sea salt
8 ounces shelled whole oysters (can use canned + liquid from can)
Freshly ground black pepper
¼ cup cream or milk (optional)
2 strips naturally cured bacon (optional)
Fresh parsley leaves, minced

Preparation

1. Heat oil in a large soup pot over medium-high heat. Add onions and sauté 2-3 minutes.

2. Add potatoes and stock. Bring to a boil.

3. Reduce heat to low, cover, and simmer until potatoes soften, 10-12 minutes.

4. With a slotted spoon, remove half the vegetables, and puree them in a food processor or blender.

5. Pour pureed vegetables back into the soup.

6. Add celery, carrots, tarragon, salt, oysters with their liquid, and pepper.

7. Increase heat to medium, and cook 7 minutes.

8. Reduce heat to low, and add cream.

9. The bacon can be either baked in the oven or cooked on the stovetop. If you prefer the oven method, preheat it to 400°F.

10. Place bacon on a baking sheet, and bake until crispy, or cook on the stovetop until crispy. Drain on paper towels and chop into bite-size pieces.

11. Taste and adjust seasoning if necessary. Serve

VEGETABLES

We all know how important it is to eat our vegetables—when they are properly prepared. Vegetables can be prepared in a variety of ways: raw, cooked, steamed, sautéed, blanched, boiled, pureed, pressed, and fermented.

Vegetables can be a delicious part of many healing diets, including a thyroid-healing diet. The cleansing effect of vegetables supports the body's detoxification systems.

If you are feeling cold all the time, as many thyroid-challenged people often are, eat more cooked vegetables and soups. If you are feeling toxic and stagnant and feel that your liver needs a break, eat more raw salads.

Remember to use the produce that is local and seasonal in your area, and eat a little combination of all types of vegetables, both cooked and raw, to help you find balance.

Mineral-Rich Mushroom Soup

Ingredients

1-2 tablespoons grass-fed butter or olive oil

3-4 shallots, peeled and minced, or 1 large onion, peeled and diced

8 ounces cremini mushrooms, wiped with a damp towel or brushed, chopped (approximately 4 cups)

4 ounces fresh shitake mushrooms, wiped with a damp towel or brushed, chopped (approximately 2 cups)

4 cups chicken stock, beef stock, veggie stock, or water

1 tablespoon fresh tarragon leaves or 1 teaspoon dried

1 teaspoon sea salt

Fresh chives, minced

Preparation

1. Heat butter in a large soup pot over medium-high heat. Add shallots, and sauté 2-3 minutes.

2. Add mushrooms, and continue sautéing 3-5 minutes.

3. Add stock, tarragon, and salt; bring to a boil.

4. Cover, reduce heat, and simmer for 5-7 minutes.

5. Remove shallots and mushrooms with a slotted spoon and puree in a food processor or blender.

6. Add pureed vegetables back into the soup and stir.

7. Taste, and adjust seasoning if needed.

8. Serve garnished with fresh chives.

Traditional Minestrone Soup

Ingredients

1 tablespoon olive oil
1 leek, white and light green parts, cleaned and chopped
3-4 cloves garlic, peeled and diced
4-5 cups bone stock (beef, chicken, or duck)
2 carrots, rinsed and sliced into ¼-inch rounds
1 celery stalk, rinsed and diced
1½ teaspoons sea salt
1 tablespoon fresh thyme leaves or 1 teaspoon dried
½ teaspoon dried oregano leaves
½ teaspoon dried rosemary leaves
½ cup elbow pasta (rice, quinoa, or semolina pasta)
1½ cups cooked cannellini beans
3-4 leaves Swiss chard, chopped
Parmigiano Reggiano cheese (optional)

Preparation

1. Heat oil in a soup pot over medium-high heat. Add leeks, and sauté 2-3 minutes.

2. Add garlic, stock, carrots, celery, salt, thyme, oregano, and rosemary.

3. Cover, and cook over medium-high heat 7-10 minutes.

4. Add pasta, beans, and Swiss chard; bring to a boil.

5. Cover, reduce heat to low, and cook an additional 8-10 minutes.

6. Serve garnished with shaved cheese.

Simple Sauerkraut

If you're feeling adventurous and want to prepare your own sauerkraut, I fully support you! It takes a little bit of time and work, but can be highly beneficial to your health. If you're not feeling up for the task, you can always purchase fermented vegetables in your local health food store. You will need two 2-quart mason jars, canning jars, or a crock for this recipe.

Ingredients

3 heads green cabbage, reserve 2 leaves and shred the rest
1½-2 tablespoons sea salt
1½ teaspoons caraway seeds
1½ teaspoons juniper berries

Preparation

1. Combine cabbage and salt in a large bowl.

2. Work the salt into the cabbage by using pressure and lightly squeezing as you work it in. Or use a mallet or something else heavy to crush the vegetable fibers.

3. The cabbage will begin releasing liquid.

4. Toss in caraway seeds and juniper berries, and mix.

5. Pack the mixture, plus all of the liquid, into the jars or a crock.

6. Firmly press a cabbage leaf on top of the mixture.

7. Make sure cabbage is completely submerged in the salty liquid.

8. Cover the mouth of the jar with cheesecloth and set on the counter, out of the sun.

9. Let the kraut ferment for 10 days
   (up to 3 months for a more sour kraut!).

10. The kraut must always be submerged in the liquid.

11. After 7-10 days, remove the top leaf and discard. Also discard any discolored cabbage.

12. Once your kraut is ready, refrigerate it. It will keep for 2-3 months.

Braised Kale with White Beans

Ingredients

1 cup chicken stock or water
1 bunch kale, rinsed and chopped into bite-size pieces
1½ cups cooked white beans (cannellini or Great Northern)
2-3 cloves garlic, peeled and thinly sliced
1 tablespoon olive oil
¼ teaspoon sea salt

Preparation

1. Place stock and kale into a deep frying pan.

2. Cook over medium-high heat until kale is wilted, 3-5 minutes.

3. Add beans, garlic, oil, and salt.

4. Toss, and cook an additional 3-5 minutes.

Steamed Winter Vegetables

Ingredients

1 leek, white and light green parts, cleaned and chopped

2 carrots, rinsed and cut into thick matchsticks

¼ head cabbage, rinsed and dried, sliced into thin strips

2-3 kale leaves, rinsed and dried, thinly sliced

2 teaspoons organic olive oil

2 pinches sea salt

Preparation

1. Place ⅓ cup water, leeks, carrots, cabbage, and kale into a sauté pan.

2. Cover, bring to a boil, and steam 2-3 minutes.

3. Uncover, and continue cooking until remaining water evaporates.

4. Add oil and salt to the vegetables. Toss to coat evenly, and remove from the heat.

Caramelized Roots

Ingredients

2-3 carrots, rinsed and chopped

2-3 parsnips, rinsed and chopped

1 daikon, rinsed and chopped

2 tablespoons olive oil or duck fat

Sea salt

Freshly ground black pepper

1 tablespoon minced fresh parsley leaves

Preparation

1. Preheat oven to 375°F.

2. Place roots into a large bowl. Add oil and toss to coat evenly.

3. Season with salt and pepper.

4. Place roots into a 9- ×13-inch baking pan, and cover tightly with aluminum foil.

5. Roast roots 35-40 minutes.

6. Uncover, and continue roasting until roots caramelize (brown or lightly blacken), 25-30 minutes.

7. Serve as a side dish, garnished with minced parsley.

Deep Root Sesame Sauté

Burdock is an underused root vegetable that helps digest fat and oil and aids in healing the skin. For those of you who are suffering from dry skin and eczema as symptoms of your thyroid condition, eat burdock at least one time per week.

Ingredients

2 burdock roots, rinsed and cut diagonally in ⅛-inch slices

3-4 carrots, rinsed and cut diagonally in ⅛-inch slices

1 tablespoon toasted sesame oil

1 tablespoon mirin rice wine

3 tablespoons shoyu or wheat-free tamari

¼ cup hulled sesame seeds, toasted

Preparation

1. Place burdocks into a frying pan and lay carrots on top.

2. Mix sesame oil, mirin, shoyu, and ⅓ cup water in a bowl, and pour over vegetables. Bring to a boil.

3. Cover, reduce heat to low, and cook until liquid evaporates, 20-25 minutes.

4. Toss with toasted sesame seeds.

Crispy Kale Chips

Ingredients

1 bunch kale, rinsed and dried
1 tablespoon olive oil
Sea salt

Preparation

1. Preheat oven to 350°F.

2. Remove kale stems (can discard or save for stir fry).

3. Rip kale leaves into bite-size pieces and place into a large bowl.

4. Season with oil. Do NOT add salt.

5. Place oiled kale onto a cookie sheet or baking tray.

6. Roast until kale is crispy, 10-12 minutes.

7. Remove from the oven, and season lightly with salt.

Spring Cobb Salad with Honey Dressing

Springtime is flower time! If you visit a farmer's market, you can usually find many varieties of edible flowers that will make your salad look bright and beautiful.

Ingredients

2 cups mixed baby greens (mizuna, mesclun, lettuces), rinsed and dried
2 pastured eggs, hard-cooked and quartered
2 ounces raw milk Cheddar cheese, cubed
1 strip naturally cured pastured bacon, cooked until crispy, chopped
¼ cup extra virgin olive oil
1 shallot, peeled and minced
2 tablespoons apple cider vinegar
2 teaspoons raw local honey
Sea salt
Freshly ground black pepper
Kale flowers or arugula flowers

Preparation

1. Place greens into a large mixing bowl.

2. Top greens with eggs, cheese, and bacon.

3. In a small bowl, whisk together oil, shallots, vinegar, and honey.

4. Season the dressing with salt and pepper to taste.

5. Drizzle dressing on top of salad.

6. Serve garnished with kale flowers.

Bone Broth Miso Soup

I encourage many of my clients who are suffering from thyroid conditions to try miso soup, especially for breakfast. Eating miso soup can help support and heal their digestive systems. As you learned in the "Healthful Foods That Are NOT So Healthful" chapter, many people are eating tofu and soy products that have not been properly prepared, which can lead to many thyroid conditions. Miso soup is the traditional preparation of soy that makes it nourishing and supportive rather than damaging to your thyroid gland.

Ingredients

4-5 inches dried alaria or wakame (sea vegetables)

5 cups Iodine-Rich Fish Stock

6-8 ounces extra firm tofu, cubed, or 6-8 ounces fish, cubed (can use both)

4 tablespoons sweet white miso or aduki bean miso

2-3 scallions, white and light green parts, rinsed and minced

Preparation

1. Reconstitute alaria in a small amount of cool water for 10-15 minutes. After it softens Drain, and discard the soaking water. Cut the alaria into thin slices.

2. Place stock, tofu, fish (if using), and alaria in a pot. Bring to a boil.

3. Reduce heat to medium-low.

4. In a small bowl, dilute miso in a small amount of warm water, and stir back into the soup.

5. Continue cooking 2-3 minutes.

6. Serve garnished with scallions.

Crisp Caesar Salad

Whenever I feel like I need a quick hit of iodine, I opt for a miso soup or a Caesar salad. The anchovies used in this dressing are rich in vitamin B12, iodine, protein, and deliciousness. Try it—you'll LOVE it!

Ingredients

2 heads Romaine lettuce, washed and chopped into bite-size pieces
1 small red onion or 1 large shallot, peeled and sliced into thin crescents
6-8 ounces grilled pastured chicken, cut into 1-inch cubes (optional)
Caesar Salad Dressing (see recipe below)
1 tablespoon grated Parmigiano Reggiano cheese

Preparation

1. Combine lettuce, onions, and chicken in a large mixing bowl.

2. Toss, and coat evenly with Caesar Salad Dressing.

3. Serve garnished with cheese.

Caesar Salad Dressing

Ingredients

⅓ cup olive oil
3-5 anchovy fillets
2-3 cloves garlic, peeled and chopped
1 tablespoon Dijon mustard
1 tablespoon mayonnaise (optional for creamier consistency)
2 tablespoons red or white wine vinegar
¼ cup freshly grated imported
Parmigiano Reggiano cheese
Sea salt
Freshly ground black pepper

Preparation

1. Combine oil, anchovies, garlic, mustard, mayonnaise, vinegar, and cheese in a food processor or blender.

2. Season with salt and pepper to taste.

Marinated Dandelion and Radish Salad

Ingredients

1 bunch dandelion greens, rinsed, dried, and chopped

8-10 red radishes, rinsed and sliced into thin half moons

3-4 scallions, white and light green parts, rinsed and chopped

¼ cup extra virgin olive oil

2 tablespoons apple cider vinegar

2 teaspoons local honey

Sea salt

Freshly ground black pepper

Preparation

1. Combine dandelion greens, radishes, and scallions in a large mixing bowl.

2. In a small bowl, whisk together oil, vinegar, and honey.

3. Season with salt and pepper.

4. Pour dressing over salad.

5. Toss, and marinate, covered, 35-40 minutes, or, for best results, overnight in the refrigerator.

6. Toss again and serve.

DESSERT!

Yes, of course dessert gets an exclamation mark! People love sweets. While you're healing your condition, I'm going to suggest that you limit the number of sweets and desserts you are eating.

Start incorporating more love and internal sweetness: loving thoughts, loving words, loving self, and loving others. Internal sweetness also includes doing activities and work that you love. When you are engaged in an activity you enjoy (singing, writing, dancing, artwork, pottery, gardening, walking in nature), the desire for sweets, and for food in general, disappears. As internal sweetness increases, the craving for external sweetness naturally diminishes.

That being said, you can still eat dessert! But please minimize the number of processed sweets as you are healing your gut and body. Go for natural sweets like sweet vegetables and fruits as often as possible. And, occasionally (not daily), treat yourself to something more indulgent. Enjoy!

Baked Stuffed Apples with Walnuts and Raisins

Ingredients

4 apples, cored
½ cup walnuts, chopped
3 tablespoons raisins
1 tablespoon honey
1 teaspoon ground cinnamon
1 dash ground cloves
1 tablespoon brown sugar (or other sugar)
2 tablespoons grass-fed butter

Preparation

1. Preheat oven to 350°F.

2. Place apples into a 9-inch square baking dish.

3. In a small bowl, combine walnuts, raisins, honey, cinnamon, cloves, sugar, and butter.

4. Stuff cored apples with walnut raisin mixture.

5. Bake apples until tender and golden, 35-40 minutes.

Gluten-Free Goji Berry Jam Dot Cookies

Ingredients

½ cup dried goji berries
½ cup unsweetened apple or black cherry juice
¾ cup granulated maple sugar
½ cup grass-fed butter
1 large egg, beaten
1 teaspoon vanilla extract
1½ cups white rice flour
½ teaspoon ground cinnamon
1 teaspoon baking powder
¼ teaspoon sea salt
Coconut oil

Preparation

1. Place goji berries in a bowl. Add fruit juice, and soak until soft, 1-2 hours.

2. Place goji berries plus juice into a saucepot. Cook over medium-high heat until goji berries burst open and the fruit reduces and thickens, 7-10 minutes.

3. Transfer to a bowl, cover, let chill in refrigerator while you prepare the cookie dough.

4. In a mixing bowl, combine maple sugar and butter.

5. Add egg and vanilla.

6. In a separate bowl, combine flour, cinnamon, baking powder, and salt.

7. Combine the wet and dry ingredients and mix well until it forms dough.

8. Transfer the dough to a work surface, and form it into a log.

9. Cover with plastic wrap and refrigerate until firm, 1-2 hours.

10. Preheat oven to 350°F. Lightly oil a cookie sheet with coconut oil.

11. Pull off pieces of the dough, and roll into two-inch balls. Place the balls on the prepared cookie sheet.

12. Flatten the cookies a little, and press an indentation in the center of the cookie with your thumb or forefinger.

13. Spoon ½ to 1 teaspoon chilled goji berries into the indentation.

14. Bake cookies until golden brown, about 12 minutes.

Apple Crumble

To make this crumble gluten-free, use oat flour, rice flour or any other gluten-free flour you would like.

Ingredients

Filling:
4 apples, cored and diced
⅓ cup apple juice
Juice of 1 lemon

Topping:
¾ cup whole grain all-purpose flour, rice flour, or oat flour
½ cup rolled oats
⅓ cup maple sugar
½ teaspoon ground allspice
¼ teaspoon sea salt
5-6 tablespoons grass-fed butter, cut into small pieces

Preparation

1. Preheat oven to 375°F.

2. Place diced apples in a 9-inch square casserole dish with apple juice and lemon juice.

3. Combine flour, oats, maple sugar, allspice, and salt in a small bowl.

4. Work butter into the flour mixture until it looks like crumbs.

5. Top apples with crumb mixture.

6. Bake until golden brown and bubbling, 40-45 minutes.

Strawberries with Cream

Ingredients

⅓ cup organic or grass-fed heavy cream

½ teaspoon vanilla extract

2 tablespoons organic powdered sugar (optional)

1 pint fresh strawberries, rinsed and patted dry

Preparation

1. In a large bowl, combine heavy cream and vanilla extract.

2. Begin whipping with a whisk.

3. Add powdered sugar and continue whisking until soft peaks form.

4. Spoon into a bowl.

5. Dip strawberries into the fresh whipped cream, and go straight to heaven.

Wild Blackberry Cobbler

Ingredients

Filling:
3 cups wild blackberries (can use store-bought), rinsed and dried
¼ cup apple juice
2 tablespoons maple sugar or other sugar
½ teaspoon vanilla extract
1 tablespoon grass-fed butter, cut into thin slices

Topping:
1½ cups all-purpose flour, rice flour, or oat flour
⅓ cup maple sugar, granulated cane juice, or other sugar
2 pinches sea salt
6-8 tablespoons grass-fed butter

Preparation

1. Preheat oven to 375°F.

2. Place berries into a 9-inch square baking dish.

3. In a small bowl or pitcher, combine apple juice with sugar and vanilla, and pour on top of berries.

4. Drop butter pieces on top of berries.

5. Place flour, maple sugar, and salt into a large mixing bowl.

6. Cut butter into ½-inch squares, and combine with dry ingredients.

7. Mix flour and butter with your hands until it resembles large crumbles.

8. Sprinkle crumbles on top of blackberries. Do not pack down.

9. Bake, uncovered, until light brown and bubbling, 35-45 minutes.

Baked Pears with Cranberry Reduction

Ingredients

4 Bosc pears
1 cup apple juice
1 cup cranberry juice
2 cinnamon sticks
6-8 whole cloves

Preparation

1. Preheat oven to 400°F.

2. Cut a thin slice off the bottom of each pear to help them stand upright.

3. Arrange the pears in a 9-inch square baking dish.

4. Pour fruit juices into the baking dish.

5. Add cinnamon sticks and cloves.

6. Roast the pears, basting every 15 minutes, until tender, brown, and puckered, approximately 1 hour and 15 minutes.

7. Transfer the pears to a serving plate.

8. Pour any remaining liquid from the baking pan into a small saucepan, and bring to a boil.

9. Reduce by half.

10. Drizzle that liquid on top of the pears.

RESOURCES

Arbor Vitae School of Traditional Herbalism
Arborvitaeny.com
646-721-5998

Claudia Keel
Herbs & Essences
Earthflower.org
Email: Claudia@earthflower.org

Richard Mandelbaum
Clinical Herbalist
Richardmandelbaum.com
Email: nyherbalist@gmail.com

Karyn Bender
Integrative Pharmacist, Herbalist, Holistic Health & Nutrition Coach,
Certified Medical Intuitive.
www.KarynBender.com

Matthew Wood
Matthewwoodherbs.com
Email: greenmedic@copper.net

Tammi Sweet
Tsweet24@hotmail.com
Heartstone Center for Earth Essentials
Heart-stone.com
info@heart-stone.com

American Herbalists Guild
Locate an Herbalist near you
Americanherbalistsguild.com
Email: office@americanherbalistsguild.com
617-520-4372

James MacLean, L.Ac.
Classical Chinese Medicine
Acupuncture & Herbal Medicine
Qispirit.com
Email: jwwm@earthlink.net
917-334-4779

Robert Peng
www.robertpeng.com
Qigong practitioner
RobertQigongSeminar@gmail.com

Master Jey Park
Vital Ki Energy Practitioner
Email: ask@vitalkienergy-jungshim.org
212-604-9595

WHERE TO PURCHASE HIGH QUALITY BULK HERBS

Woodland Essence
Herbal tinctures
Woodlandessence.com
Email: woodland@ntcnet.com

Walker Herbs
Herbal tinctures
Walkerherbs.com
Email: jmzsenior@gmail.com

Flower Power
Bulk Herbs
Flowerpower.net
406 East 9th Street
New York, NY 10009

Mountain Rose Herbs
Bulk Herbs
Mountainroseherbs.com
support@mountainroseherbs.co
800-879-3337

Maine Seaweed
Larch Hanson
Theseaweedman.com
Email: hanson.larch@gmail.com
207-546-2875

Island Herbs
Ryan Drum
Ryandrum.com

Maine Coast Sea Vegetables
Seaveg.com
info@seaveg.com
207-412-0094

FIND THE BEST QUALITY FOOD

Localharvest.org
Eatwild.org
Seafoodwatch.org
Eatwellguide.com

RECIPE INDEX

CPSIA information can be obtained
at www.ICGtesting.com
Printed in the USA
BVOW11s0819090118

504785BV00008B/13/P